TRA

2ⁿᵈ edition

TRANSFUSION SCIENCE

2nd edition

J. Overfield

Division of Health Science, School of Biology, Chemistry and Health Science, Manchester Metropolitan University, Manchester, UK

M. Dawson

Centre for Learning and Teaching, Manchester Metropolitan University, Manchester, UK

and

D. Hamer

Pathology Department, Royal Bolton Hospital, Bolton, UK

Scion

Second edition © Scion Publishing Ltd, 2008

ISBN 978 1 904842 40 8

First edition published in 1999 by Butterworth Heinemann (ISBN 0 7506 3415 4)

A CIP catalogue record for this book is available from the British Library.

Scion Publishing Limited
Bloxham Mill, Barford Road, Bloxham, Oxfordshire OX15 4FF
www.scionpublishing.com

Important Note from the Publisher

The information contained within this book was obtained by Scion Publishing Limited from sources believed by us to be reliable. However, while every effort has been made to ensure its accuracy, no responsibility for loss or injury whatsoever occasioned to any person acting or refraining from action as a result of information contained herein can be accepted by the authors or publishers.

Typeset by Phoenix Photosetting, Chatham, Kent, UK
Printed by Gutenberg Press Ltd, Malta

Contents

Preface

We are very pleased to write the second edition of this text, particularly as there have been a number of significant changes in transfusion science since the first edition in 1999.

The potential risk of prion-related disease transmission was just beginning to be realized and has now become recognized as highly significant, along with many other serious hazards of transfusion. Transfusion science has become increasingly important in the light of increasing knowledge due to extensive research using the analytical tools which have become available in recent years.

A new chapter (13) has been written to introduce the student to the current applications of emerging techniques in transfusion science. Immunotechniques, using flow cytometry, and molecular biology techniques have had a significant impact on transfusion practice and we have described these in some detail.

Many sections have been revised. In Chapter 8, the section on red cell destruction has been extended, and the inclusion of platelet immune disorders as well as haemolytic anaemias is new. Chapter 9 describes the need for leucodepletion and introduces methods for pathogen reduction. Chapter 10 focuses on gel techniques and reviews current practice in blood group serology. New nomenclature for blood group genes has been adopted in Chapters 5, 6 and 7. Chapter 11 covers recent legislation for quality aspects of transfusion in the United Kingdom.

Further key changes include the use of case studies to illustrate concepts, colour photographs to aid understanding and an extended contents list to help locate the material more easily. Self-assessment questions and learning outcomes are also provided.

Transfusion science issues are rapidly changing and the student is advised to be aware of the importance of constantly updating current practices to meet the needs which arise from environmental issues in society. Although we have remained focused on current practice in the United Kingdom, we have retained awareness that this text has been adopted for students of transfusion science worldwide.

Thanks are given to Jonathan Ray (Scion Publishing Ltd), Hazel Powell (Manchester Blood Centre) for valuable feedback and Mick Hoult (Manchester Metropolitan University) for providing many of the figures and images. Special thanks go to our families for their patience and support, and finally, to our students for providing the motivation to write this book.

Joyce Overfield, Maureen Dawson and David Hamer
July 2007

Preface to first edition

The science of transfusion is a constantly growing and changing subject. In recent years, new diseases have arisen which may be transmissable by blood and its components. Even as this book has been in progress, changes have occurred in society and our environment that future biomedical scientists in the transfusion world cannot ignore. Despite these impacts, the transfusion service strives to continue to provide safe products. In addition, much of the underlying learning basis for the student remains constant. For example, antigen and antibody structures and interactions, the mechanism of action of complement and autoimmune haemolysis are relatively well known. Changes are taking place in the field of transplantation and we have attempted to introduce students to the issues and requirements surrounding this important area as treatments continue to develop.

In this volume, we hope to introduce medical and biomedical science students and scientists to basic principles in transfusion, whilst also increasing awareness of current issues and developments. We believe that this book will provide those who read it with a good basis on which to build their understanding of transfusion service.

We are grateful to Vin Sakalas at the Manchester Blood Centre for helpful advice on current issues with regard to blood products. Thanks also go to Chris Pallister and the staff at Butterworth-Heinemann for their advice and support and the co-authors would like to thank D. Hamer for the computer-generated figures. Finally, we would like to thank our families for their patience.

J. Overfield, M. Dawson and D. Hamer

Abbreviations

AA	amino acid	CPDA	citrate phosphate dextrose adenine
ADCC	antibody-dependent cellular cytotoxicity	CR	complement receptor
AGT	antiglobulin test	CRP	C-reactive protein
AHG	anti-human globulin	CTH	ceramide trihexose
AIHA	autoimmune haemolytic anaemia	CTL	cytotoxic T lymphocytes
		CVF	cobra venom factor
AITP	autoimmune thrombocytopenic purpura	DAF	decay accelerating factor
		DARC	Duffy antigen receptor for chemokines
ALL	acute lymphoblastic leukaemia	DAT	direct antiglobulin test
		DIC	disseminated intravascular coagulation
AML	acute myelogenous leukaemia	DMSO	dimethyl sulphoxide
APC	antigen-presenting cells	DNA	deoxyribonucleic acid
ARDS	adult respiratory distress syndrome	DPG	diphosphoglycerate
		EBV	Epstein–Barr virus
AS-PCR	allele-specific PCR	EDTA	ethylenediaminetetra-acetic acid
BMT	bone marrow transplant		
BPO	benzylpenicilloyl	EPO	erythropoietin
BSA	bovine serum albumin	Fab	fragment antigen-binding
BSE	bovine spongiform encephalopathy		
		FC-PIFT	flow cytometry by platelet indirect immunofluorescence test
CAM	cell adhesion molecule		
CD	cluster of differentiation		
CDH	ceramide dihexose	FFP	fresh frozen plasma
cDNA	complementary DNA	FITC	fluoroscein isothiocyanate
CDR	complementarity determining region		
		FMH	foetomaternal haemorrhage
CGD	chronic granulomatous disease		
		FSC	forward scatter
CJD	Creutzfeldt–Jakob disease	Fuc	L-fucose
CLL	chronic lymphocytic leukaemia	Gal	D-galactose
		GalNAc	N-acetyl-galactosamine
CLT	chemiluminescence test	G-CSF	granulocyte-colony stimulating factor
CMI	cell-mediated immunity		
CML	chronic myelogenous leukaemia	GM-CSF	granulocyte-macrophage colony stimulating factor
CMV	cytomegalovirus	GP	glycoprotein

GPA	glycophorin A	MASP	mannose binding lectin associated proteases
GPB	glycophorin B	MBL	mannose-binding lectin
GVHD	graft-versus-host disease	MCA	middle cerebral artery
HAV	hepatitis A virus	MCV	mean cell volume
Hb	haemoglobin	MHC	major histocompatibility complex
HbA	haemoglobin in adult red cells	MIRL	membrane inhibitor of reacting lysis
HbF	haemoglobin in foetal cells	MLR	mixed lymphocyte reaction
HBV	hepatitis B virus	mRNA	messenger RNA
HCDM	human cell differentiation molecules	NAITP	neonatal alloimmune thrombocytopenic purpura
Hct	haematocrit	NAT	nucleic acid testing
HCV	hepatitis C virus	NHFTR	non-haemolytic febrile transfusion reactions
HDN	haemolytic disease of the newborn	NIS-AGT	normal ionic strength antiglobulin test
HIV	human immunodeficiency virus	NK cells	natural killer cells
HLA	human leucocyte antigen	PBL	peripheral blood lymphocytes
HLDA	human leucocyte differentiation antigen	PBSC	peripheral blood stem cell
HPA	human platelet antigen	PBSCT	peripheral blood stem cell transplantation
HSC	haemopoietic stem cells	PCH	paroxysmal cold haemoglobinuria
HSCT	haemopoietic stem cell transplants	PCR	polymerase chain reaction
HTLV	human T cell leukemia virus	PCV	packed cell volume
HTR	haemolytic transfusion reaction	PE	phycoerythrin
IAT	indirect antiglobulin technique	PEG	polyethylene glycol
IFN	interferon	PIG A	phosphatidylinositol glycan A
Ig	immunoglobulin	PMN	polymorphonuclear leucocytes
IHA	immune haemolytic anaemia	PNH	paroxysmal nocturnal haemoglobinuria
IL	interleukin	PPP	platelet-poor plasma
LGL	large granular lymphocytes	PRP	platelet-rich plasma
LIS-AGT	low ionic strength antiglobulin test	PTP	post-transfusion purpura
LISS	low ionic strength solutions	RCF	relative centrifugal force
MAC	membrane attack complex	RE	reticuloendothelial
MALT	mucosa-associated lymphoid tissue		

RFLP	restriction fragment length polymorphism	SSOP	sequence-specific oligonucleotide probing
RIC	reduced intensity conditioning	SSP	sequence specific priming
RID	radial immunodiffusion	TC	cytotoxic precursor T lymphocytes
RMM	relative molecular mass		
RNA	ribonucleic acid	TCR	T cell receptor
SABRE	Serious Adverse Blood Reactions and Events	TH	helper T lymphocytes
		TNF	tumour necrosis factor
SAGM	saline, containing adenine, glucose and mannitol	TNF-α	tumour necrosis factor alpha
		TPH	transplacental haemorrhage
SCID	severe combined immunodeficiency disease	TPHA	*Treponema pallidum* haemagglutination assay
SHOT	Serious Hazards of Transfusion	TRALI	transfusion related acute lung injury
SLE	systemic lupus erythematosus	tRNA	transfer RNA
		vCJD	variant Creutzfeldt–Jakob disease
SNP	single nucleotide polymorphism		
SRID	single radial immunodiffusion	VP	viral peptide
		vWd	von Willebrand disease
SSC	side scatter	vWf	von Willebrand factor

Colour plates

Chapter 5. Introduction to blood groups: the ABO blood group system

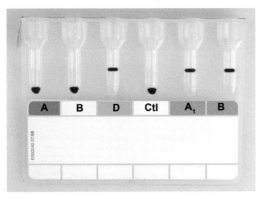

(a)

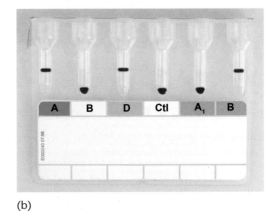

(b)

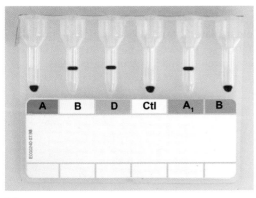

(c)

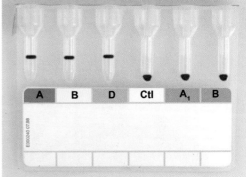

(d)

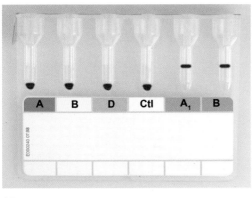

(e)

Colour plate 1. Gel card technology illustrating ABO blood group results.

Gel cards contain the following reagents (from left to right): anti-A, anti-B, anti-D. Patient's red cells are added to the first three microtubes. Three microtubes contain gel only, for a control (Ctl), and the addition of A₁ and B red cells with patient's serum.

(a) O Rh D positive
(b) A Rh D positive
(c) B Rh D positive
(d) AB Rh D positive
(e) O Rh D negative

Chapter 8. Immune and autoimmune haematology disorders

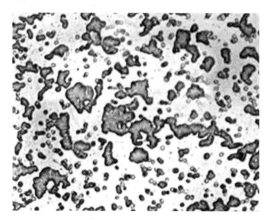

Colour plate 2. Red cell agglutination seen in the peripheral blood smear of a patient with immune haemolytic anaemia (Romanowsky stain).

Chapter 9. Blood products and components

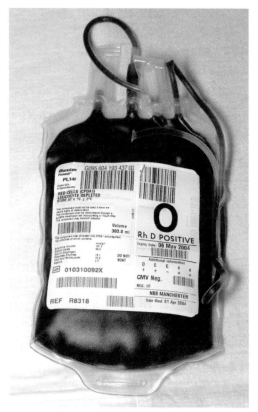

Colour plate 3. (a) A unit of red cells – note the information provided by bar codes. (b) A unit of fresh frozen plasma. (c) A unit of platelets.

(a)

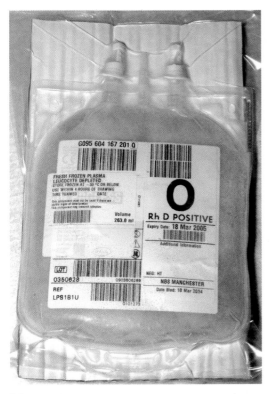

(b)

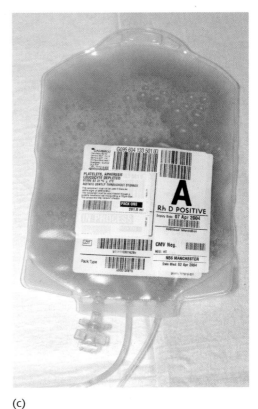

(c)

Chapter 10. Haemagglutination and blood grouping methods

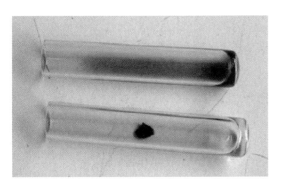

Colour plate 4. Free red cells (top) and agglutinated red cells (bottom) by tube technique.

The immune system

Learning objectives
After studying this chapter you should be able to:

- Discuss the differences between non-specific and specific immune defences
- Outline the roles of complement, interferons and cytokines in non-specific defences
- Describe the cells of the non-specific defences and outline their roles
- Describe the major features of inflammation and the acute phase response
- Discuss the differences between humoral and cell-mediated specific immunity
- Define the terms: immunogen, antigen, epitope and hapten
- Discuss the roles of B and T lymphocytes in specific immune responses

1.1 IMMUNOLOGY AND TRANSFUSION SCIENCE

Immunology is the study of the physiological mechanisms which defend the body against infection by microorganisms. It includes a study of the organs, tissues, cells and macromolecules involved both in preventing the entry of microorganisms to the body and in eliminating microorganisms which do gain entry. An essential feature of the immune system is the ability to distinguish between 'self' and 'non-self' so that the response is targeted at material foreign to the body, and not its own components.

Knowledge of the immune system is essential to the transfusion scientist for a number of reasons. First, the immune response which distinguishes self from non-self is also responsible for the consequences of the transfusion of mismatched blood (Chapter 11). Similarly, it is the immune system which causes diseases such as haemolytic disease of the newborn (HDN) due to incompatibilities between maternal and foetal blood groups, while immune system dysregulation is responsible for autoimmune disorders such as autoimmune haemolytic anaemia (Chapter 8). Knowledge of the immune system also explains the need for close matching of donated stem cells to a potential recipient in order to prevent the occurrence of graft-versus-host disease (GVHD; Chapter 12).

Immunological components other than blood may be transfused, or may be measured and/or used in the transfusion science laboratory, for example, antibodies (Chapter 2) and complement (Chapter 3). In addition, pathologists and clinicians have been able to make use of products of the immune system in many different ways. Antibodies, for example, are used for developing highly sensitive assays and cytokines are used therapeutically. This chapter will give an outline of the major components of the immune system and how these components interact to protect the body from infectious disease.

1.2 THE IMMUNE SYSTEM

The bodies of multicellular animals are constantly threatened by the multitude of microorganisms which exist outside them. Many of these microorganisms are potentially pathogenic, that is, they can cause disease in various ways. Bacteria, for example, may produce toxins while viruses enter living cells where they replicate, eventually causing cell death. Protozoal parasites may subvert the normal physiological mechanisms in many different ways. For example, *Plasmodium,* the malarial parasite, lyses red cells and causes glomerulonephritis and damage to small blood vessels. Finally, multicellular parasites such as nematodes may damage the tissues and organs they inhabit at different stages of their complex life cycles.

All multicellular animals have defence mechanisms to keep out potentially harmful microorganisms or to remove them from the body once they have entered. The set of defence mechanisms is known as the **immune system**. The human immune system is essentially the same as the immune system of other mammals and similar to that of other higher vertebrates. This immune system is able to distinguish between the cells and macromolecules that make up the body and those that do not. In other words, the immune system is able to distinguish between **self** and **non-self**.

1.3 TWO TYPES OF IMMUNE DEFENCE

Immunological defences are usually classified into two kinds, depending on what exactly is being recognized. For example, some defences are **non-specific** and these are targeted at any material which is foreign to the body, including substances such as wood splinters, as well as microorganisms. This is one of the reasons why materials used in medical prostheses, such as artificial hip joints, have to be thoroughly tested before use. If unsuitable, they may trigger the body's defence mechanisms and induce an unacceptable inflammatory reaction. Non-specific defences are available immediately an organism enters the body and they constitute a first line of defence.

As well as non-specific defences, there is a series of **specific** immune defences in which cells and macromolecules are able to recognize not only individual microorganisms, but also the particular proteins or glycoproteins which make up that microorganism. The specific immune system is essential for the maintenance of health because, once activated, it can result in **immunity** to a microorganism. A specific immune response may take several days to produce its effect, especially following a first encounter with the foreign cells or proteins. In transfusion, this may explain why a haemolytic reaction to foreign red blood cells may sometimes occur several days after the transfusion has taken place. It is important to remember, though, that the distinctions between non-specific and specific immunological defences can become blurred because there are so many interactions between the two. For example, non-specific cells such as macrophages are often required to initiate specific immunity and, once activated, the products of this system bring about removal of microorganisms, for the most part by stimulating the non-specific defences.

1.4 NON-SPECIFIC DEFENCES

A list of some of the important non-specific defences is shown in *Table 1.1*. Some of these defences which are relevant to transfusion science are discussed below.

Table 1.1 The major non-specific immunological defences

Defence	Example
Structural barriers	Skin, mucosal membranes
Acidity	Lactic acid in sweat; HCl in stomach
Proteins	Complement; lysozyme; interferons
Phagocytic cells	Monocytes; macrophages; neutrophilic polymorphonuclear leucocytes (neutrophils); eosinophilic polymorphonuclear leucocytes (eosinophils)
Non-phagocytic cells	Natural killer (NK) cells; basophilic polymorphonuclear leucocytes (basophils)
Physiological responses	Inflammation; the acute phase response

Complement

Complement is the name given to a set of proteins found in fresh plasma, which have a variety of important immunological roles. These include causing lysis of bacteria and yeasts, and stimulating phagocytosis and inflammation. Complement proteins are present in an inactive form in plasma but they may become activated by the microorganism itself (alternative and lectin pathways), or by antibodies bound to a microorganism (classical pathway). This is discussed in detail in Chapter 3. Complement can also be activated by other proteins such as C-reactive protein (CRP) and mannose binding lectin (MBL), which are produced during an infection by cells in the liver.

Interferons

People who have an active viral infection are commonly resistant to infection with another virus, a phenomenon, known as 'viral interference', which was first described by Jenner in 1804. In 1957, Isaacs and Lindenmann showed that cultured fragments of chick embryo chorioallantoic membrane deliberately infected with influenza virus secreted a substance into the culture medium which could interfere with viral replication. This substance was called interferon.

An interferon (IFN) is now defined as a protein which 'exerts virus non-specific anti-viral activity at least in homologous cells through cellular metabolic processes involving the synthesis of both RNA and protein' (Interferon Nomenclature Committee, 1980). Thus, IFNs are not directly anti-viral but act to prevent viral infection by inducing healthy cells to produce enzymes which inhibit replication of viral nucleic acid and production of viral protein. There are three major families of interferons: IFN-α, -β and -γ. IFN-α and -β are both produced by virus-infected cells while IFN-γ, discovered by Wheelock in 1965, is produced by cells of the specific immune system in response to any agent, whether bacterium, virus or foreign protein, which stimulates that system.

In the 1970s, it was shown that IFN-α could cause regression of some animal tumours and could inhibit the growth of cultured cancer cells. Since then, IFNs have been tested extensively in cancer patients. They are used therapeutically in a number of diseases (see *Box 1.1*).

Box 1.1   Interferons in therapy

Interest in the potential of IFNs as anti-cancer agents led to the testing of various forms of interferon across a range of cancers. This process was enhanced by the ability to produce recombinant proteins in bacteria such as *Escherichia coli* as well as in cultured eukaryotic cells. IFN-α2a is a recombinant protein containing 165 amino acid residues and produced in *E. coli*. It is used to treat hairy cell leukaemia, Philadelphia chromosome-positive chronic myelogenous leukaemia (CML) and AIDS-related Kaposi's sarcoma. IFN-α2b, which differs in only one amino acid from IFN-α2a, is also used to treat hairy cell leukaemia and malignant melanoma, an aggressive form of skin cancer with a high rate of recurrence. Patients are treated for several weeks after surgery, to help prevent the tumour recurring. IFNs may also be used to treat diseases other than cancer. For example, IFN-α2a and IFN-α2b are used to treat chronic viral hepatitis. IFN-β1a, a recombinant form of natural IFN-β, was introduced in 1996 for treating relapsing forms of multiple sclerosis. This IFN has been shown to decrease the number of relapses in these patients as well as the likelihood of progression. IFN-γ1b, a recombinant form of natural IFN-γ, has been shown to reduce the number of serious infections in patients with chronic granulomatous disease, an immunodeficiency disorder characterized by defective phagocytic cells.

IFNs are examples of a very broad family of proteins known as **cytokines**. Because this term will be used frequently in discussing the immune system and transfusion, this is probably a good place in which to define it.

Cytokines

Cytokines are proteins secreted by cells which bind to cell surface receptors on other cells and stimulate particular activities in them. Cytokines act at low concentrations (e.g. pg ml^{-1}) and will stimulate only those cells which have receptors for them. Depending on the cytokine and the cell being stimulated, the induced activity might be, for example, cell growth and/or differentiation, synthesis of individual proteins, increased expression of cell surface macromolecules, etc. The immune response is regulated by cytokines, several of which will be mentioned in this chapter. Some cytokines are now used therapeutically. One of the first to be used was interleukin (IL)-2, which has been used to treat renal cancer and melanoma. Granulocyte-colony stimulating factor (G-CSF) has been used to promote the production of haemopoeitic stem cells for stem cell transplants (see Chapter 12). Other cytokines have been implicated in disease processes, for example, there is evidence for the involvement of tumour necrosis factor alpha (TNF-α) in the development of septic shock, cerebral malaria and in the pathology of autoimmune disorders such as rheumatoid arthritis. In such cases, cytokine antagonists, such as antibodies to TNF, may be useful in treatment. Cytokines may also have pathological consequences in transfusion. For example, they may 'leak' from white blood cells in donated whole blood and can cause damage to tissues of the recipient and this is one of the reasons for transfusing leucodepleted blood, which is blood with the leucocytes removed, rather than whole blood (see Chapter 11)

Cells of the non-specific defences

All of the leucocytes in the blood have a role in the immune system. The leucocytes are classified into two groups: **polymorphonuclear leucocytes**

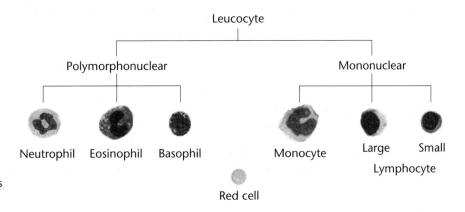

Figure 1.1
Different types of leucocyte.

(PMN), previously known as **granulocytes,** have a nucleus which is lobed, and **mononuclear leucocytes (MN)** have a nucleus which is more rounded (see *Fig. 1.1*). Three types of PMN are found in the blood: the **neutrophil,** the **basophil** and the **eosinophil.** Similarly, three types of mononuclear cells: **small lymphocytes, large granular lymphocytes (LGL)** and **monocytes** can also be found. The normal range for these cells in adult blood is shown in *Table 1.2*.

Table 1.2 Differential counts of blood leucocytes in adult Caucasians

Cell	Count ($\times 10^9$/l)
Total leucocytes	4–11
Neutrophils	2–7.5
Eosinophils	0.03–0.06
Basophils	0.02–0.29
Lymphocytes (small and large)	1.3–3.5
Monocytes	0.2–0.8

Polymorphonuclear leucocytes

The most abundant PMN, and the most easily recognized leucocyte, is the neutrophil, which makes up between 40% and 80% of the total blood leucocytes in adults. **Neutrophils** (see *Fig. 1.1*) are often called inflammatory cells because they are the first cells to arrive at a site of inflammation. Neutrophils have a nucleus which typically has between three and seven lobes. Within the cytoplasm, several types of granule can be seen. These include the azurophil granules, which contain the enzyme myeloperoxidase, as well as specific granules that contain the protein lactoferrin, and small storage granules. All the granules contain lysozyme. The neutrophil is a phagocytic cell and is highly efficient at ingesting bacteria, especially if they are coated with antibody or complement. Neutrophils are produced in the bone marrow and released into the blood, where they circulate for around 24 hours. After this time, the cell dies and is removed by other phagocytic cells, chiefly monocytes in the blood and macrophages in the spleen. The number of neutrophils in the blood increases in the few hours after an infection has become established. This is because the bone marrow is stimulated by the cytokines IL-1, TNF-α and IL-6, to release neutrophil reserves.

Neutrophils have several mechanisms for killing ingested bacteria, as shown in *Table 1.3*. Although neutrophils are able to ingest uncoated bacteria, binding to bacteria which have been coated with antibody and/or complement actually stimulates uptake and the various bactericidal mechanisms. The promotion of phagocytosis in this way is known as **opsonization.**

Table 1.3 Bactericidal mechanisms in neutrophils

Location	Mechanism
Cytoplasmic granules (lysosomes) containing hydrolytic enzymes	Primary lysosomes fuse with the phagocytic vacuoles and release these enzymes onto the bacterium
Mitochondria and azurophilic granules	A respiratory burst following ingestion of bacteria results in the production of hydrogen peroxide. Hydrogen peroxide is then converted to hypochlorite in the presence of chloride ions and the enzyme myeloperoxidase. Both hydrogen peroxide and hypochlorite have considerable anti-bacterial properties.
Myeloperoxidase-positive granules	Low molecular weight proteins known as defensins are found in these granules. These proteins attack the bacterial membrane, rendering it permeable.
Myeloperoxidase-negative granules	These contain lactoferrin, which sequesters free iron, inhibiting the growth of bacteria
Cytosol	Bacterial infection stimulates the action of nitric oxide synthase, which results in the production of nitric oxide

Basophils (see *Fig. 1.1*) make up only a small percentage of the blood leucocytes: generally less than 2% (see *Table 1.2*). The term *basophil* refers to the fact that the granules in the cytoplasm take up basic stains, such as toluidine blue. Basophils have a bi-lobed nucleus and very prominent cytoplasmic granules which contain a number of pharmacologically active chemicals. These include histamine, which dilates blood vessels and increases their permeability, heparin, which inhibits blood clotting, chemotactic factors which attract neutrophils and eosinophils, and a protease which degrades the basement membrane of blood vessels.

A cell with similarities to the blood basophils can be found in solid tissues. This cell is the **mast cell** and it has cytoplasmic granules with contents similar to those found in the basophil. Mast cells are found in several solid tissues including the skin, the mucosal membranes and epithelia of the respiratory, genitourinary and gastrointestinal tracts, and in the connective tissue of a variety of internal organs. The role of mast cells and basophils is to trigger the process of inflammation, a non-specific defence reaction to tissue injury. Though non-specific, the inflammatory process can be stimulated by antibodies, as will be discussed in Chapter 2.

Eosinophils (see *Fig. 1.1*) usually constitute less than 2% of the blood leucocytes. Like the basophils they have a highly granular cytoplasm. Unlike the basophil, however, the granules contain highly basic proteins which readily take up acidic stains such as eosin. Although eosinophils have been shown to be phagocytic cells, this role is probably a minor one. The major role of the eosinophil is to assist in the elimination of multicellular parasites such as tapeworms and nematodes. Eosinophils first bind to the surface of the worm, often through antibody, and then expel their granular proteins onto the worm surface. Eosinophils may leave the blood by migration between the endothelial cells of the blood vessel walls. They particularly migrate into an area in which mast cells have degranulated, releasing eosinophil chemotactic factors. Some cytokines, such as IL-5, increase the number and activation state of eosinophils.

Mononuclear leucocytes

Mononuclear leucocytes constitute approximately 30% of the blood leucocytes. The monocytes and the large granular lymphocytes are non-specific cells while the small lymphocytes are responsible for the specific immune response.

Monocytes comprise approximately 5% of the blood leucocytes. They have a characteristic indented, often horse-shoe-shaped nucleus and a granular cytoplasm (see *Fig. 1.1*). Monocytes in the blood may be regarded as cell 'in transit'. They are produced in the bone marrow, circulate in the blood for 8 hours and then migrate to the solid tissues where they develop into **macrophages**.

Macrophages may be 'fixed' in tissues or they may wander in an amoeboid fashion throughout the tissues (see *Table 1.4*). Organs which have an especially high content of macrophages include the spleen, the lungs, the liver, the lymph nodes and the tonsils. Monocytes and macrophages, wherever located, form the **mononuclear phagocytic system**, otherwise known as the **reticulo-endothelial system**, which clears foreign material from tissues by phagocytosis. Like the neutrophil, these cells bind readily to complement and antibody-coated material, favouring opsonization. Macrophages in particular are highly active phagocytes with a range of killing mechanisms similar to the neutrophil. Macrophages are activated by several cytokines, particularly IFN-γ, which is produced by some types of small lymphocyte. In addition, when stimulated appropriately they produce a range of cytokines, including IL-1, IL-6 and IL-8 and TNF-α. Secretion of these cytokines is stimulated following phagocytosis, especially of microorganisms such as bacteria. IL-1 and IL-6, together with TNF-α, are known to be responsible for bringing about the **acute phase response**, which is an early non-specific response to infection. IL-8 is a potent chemotactic factor for neutrophils and is one of a group of cytokines known as chemoattractant cytokines or **chemokines**.

Table 1.4 The mononuclear phagocytic system (reticuloendothelial system)

Fixed tissue macrophages	Mobile macrophages
Kupffer cells (liver)	Spleen
Alveolar macrophages (lungs)	Lymph nodes
Histiocytes (connective tissue)	Tonsils
Mesangial cells (kidney)	
Microglial cells (brain)	

As well as clearing foreign material from the body, macrophages also remove old and dying cells, such as neutrophils. These cells die after approximately 24 hours by genetically programmed self-destruction, a process known as **apoptosis** (see *Box 1.2*). Macrophages are able to detect cells undergoing apoptosis and remove them. In the spleen, macrophages remove effete red blood cells from the circulation. Complement is also involved in this process.

Finally, monocytes and macrophages are also involved in triggering the specific immune system. They 'process' foreign material so that it can be recognized by certain types of small lymphocyte; in other words, they act as **antigen-presenting cells (APC)**.

Box 1.2 How cells die

When cells are 'killed' through a toxic environmental agent, or perhaps through lack of oxygen to the tissue (anoxia), or loss of blood supply (ischaemia), they die through a process known as necrosis. Death by necrosis is somewhat 'messy' because the cell contents leak out into the surrounding tissue and can stimulate inflammation. Death of phagocytic cells by necrosis is also dangerous, because the hydrolytic enzymes they contain could cause considerable damage to the tissues surrounding the dead cell. In contrast to necrosis, most cell death is brought about by a much 'tidier', programmed method called apoptosis. Apoptosis involves rapid fragmentation of cellular DNA and subsequent fragmentation of the cell into membrane-bound apoptotic bodies which are eventually removed by phagocytes. The genetic control of this system is now being unravelled and may prove useful in the treatment of cancer. One such gene is the *TP53* gene which encodes a protein, p53, that suppresses the growth of tumours by inducing apoptosis in damaged cells.

Large granular lymphocytes (LGL) make up between 5% and 10% of the blood leucocytes. These cells have a rounded nucleus and a granular cytoplasm (see *Fig. 1.1*). They represent a mixed population of cells in terms of function. Some LGL function as natural killer (NK) cells, which have a role in anti-viral immunity because they kill virus-infected cells. NK cells are not phagocytes but kill by releasing proteins onto the target cell which perforate the cell membrane and may induce apoptosis of the infected cell. Although they do not recognize a particular virus, they help to prevent viral replication by destroying the cell in which it is replicating. NK cells may also have a role in destroying cancer cells as they arise in the body. Some LGL are also known to be able to kill cells that are coated with antibody in a process known as antibody-dependent cellular cytotoxicity (ADCC). This function is discussed in Chapter 2.

1.5 NON-SPECIFIC RESPONSES TO TISSUE DAMAGE AND INFECTION

A microorganism or other foreign material which breaches the external barriers such as the skin and mucosal membranes is subject to attack by various non-specific proteins and cells. This attack takes place in the two responses known as **inflammation** and the **acute phase response.**

Inflammation

Inflammation is a rapid and local response which is triggered initially by tissue damage. Such a rapid response is often referred to as acute inflammation, to distinguish it from the chronic inflammation which may occur if an infection persists at the site of damage. Acute inflammation is characterized by reddening, swelling, heat and pain at the damaged site. Anyone who has ever scratched their skin, or had a blister caused by badly fitting shoes will be familiar with these symptoms. Inflammation is initiated by the release of histamine from mast cells in the damaged area. Histamine stimulates dilation of blood vessels, contributing to the reddening of the damaged area and local 'heat'. Endothelial cells lining the blood vessels may contract away from each other so that plasma flows between them, into the damaged tissue. Neutrophils may also move across the blood vessel walls by first adhering to the endothelial cells, rolling over them, and migrating in the gaps between them and into the damaged area. This process is facilitated by the expression of **cell adhesion molecules (CAM)** on the endothelial cells, which bind to ligands on the neutrophils and *vice versa*. The process of inflammation serves to dilute out any harmful substance which may have entered damaged tissue and to initiate its removal by promoting the influx of neutrophils into the inflamed site.

The acute phase response

The acute phase response occurs within hours of exposure to microorganisms, though it may also be induced following extensive tissue damage such as burns to the skin or as the result of a transfusion reaction. The acute phase response is a systemic response in which a variety of organ systems, including the brain, the bone marrow, the liver, muscles and the blood are affected. The acute phase response is brought about by cytokines released by monocytes and macrophages. These cells release IL-1, IL-6 and TNF-α, which together induce a number of effects (see *Table 1.5*) There are notable changes in the composition of the blood during an acute phase response, including an increase in neutrophils, increases in free amino acid concentrations and increases in a number of defence proteins known as the **acute phase proteins**. One of the most well known of these proteins is **C-reactive protein (CRP)**. This protein is present at concentrations less than 0.11 mg per 100 ml of blood (0.11 mg dl^{-1}) prior to an acute phase response; thereafter its synthesis increases 100–1000-fold. It is a protein which can bind to certain bacteria and cause their destruction by activating complement. Levels of CRP may be elevated in inflammation generally, even if the inflammation is unrelated to infection. Thus, elevated CRP may be a risk factor for heart disease.

The effects of the acute phase response are beneficial, even if they may not always appear to be (e.g. fever, drowsiness). However, many effects of

Table 1.5 Physiological changes during an acute phase response

Physiological change	Biological significance
Fever	Increase in body temperature may inhibit the growth of bacteria and favour the development of specific immunity
Increased drowsiness	Possibly conserving energy
Loss of appetite	People often lose weight during an infectious illness, even though they have a higher nutritional requirement because of the increased protein synthesis taking place. During chronic infection, this weight loss may be highly significant
Increase in protein content in the blood	This represents increases in the acute phase proteins that are synthesized in the liver
Increased amino acid content of blood	These amino acids are derived from the breakdown of muscle protein. The amino acids are used to synthesize the acute phase proteins
Increased number of neutrophils in the blood	These are released from reserves in the bone marrow
Decreased blood zinc and iron levels	Removal inhibits the growth of bacteria
Loss of muscle tissue	The liver is supplied with amino acids to support the production of acute phase proteins. These amino acids are provided by the proteolytic breakdown of muscle tissue. This contributes to the severe 'wasting' of muscles (a condition known as **cachexia**), which can occur in chronic infections

the acute phase response have the potential to be harmful if an infection is prolonged. One example might be the severe weight loss, or **cachexia**, that may result from chronic infections such as tuberculosis. In the event of an acute phase response following a transfusion reaction, the effects are inappropriate since no infectious agent is present, and the symptoms of the acute phase response may increase the discomfort for the patient.

Inflammation and the acute phase response are very much interlinked, as indeed are all immunological responses. A chronic infection will result in a prolonged acute phase response and the long-term production of molecules which also stimulate inflammation.

1.6 THE SPECIFIC IMMUNE RESPONSE

The specific immune response allows the development of true 'immunity' to an infectious agent. Because true immunity can only develop after exposure to the microorganism (or a 'harmless' vaccine created from the microorganism), the response is often called '**acquired**'. For example, an individual who has had measles is very unlikely to get that disease again, even though they may be exposed to the virus on numerous occasions during their lifetime.

During the course of an infection such as measles, two types of specific immunity are activated. These are **humoral immunity** and **cell-mediated immunity**.

Humoral immunity involves the production of **antibodies**. These are glycoproteins, found in the plasma, lymph and body secretions such as saliva, tears, mucus and milk. Antibodies are specific to the microorganism which induced them (the **immunogen**). They have specific binding sites which allow them to bind to molecular configurations, known as **epitopes**, on the immunogen. Antibodies bind to the immunogen, marking it for destruction (see Chapter 2) by complement, phagocytes and NK cells. Antibodies also stimulate inflammation, a process which brings more phagocytes into the area.

Antibodies are produced by cells in lymphoid tissues. They are released into the lymph and eventually reach the blood.

Cell-mediated immunity (CMI) involves the specific elimination of microorganisms by cells of the immune system. This may be brought about in two ways: first, there is the production of **cytotoxic cells** capable of killing any cell infected with the microorganism which induced them. Cytotoxic cells are especially important in anti-viral immunity because viruses are obligate intracellular parasites. Destroying infected cells inhibits the virus from replicating, while antibody can 'mop up' any virus released from dead cells. Cytotoxic cells are specific, which means they will recognize and kill cells only if they recognize the virus which is infecting them. For example, cytotoxic cells induced by a measles virus will not kill cells infected with rubella virus and *vice versa*. This is in contrast to NK cells, which recognize an infected cell, rather than the virus. A second type of killing in CMI is indirect, and is mediated by cells of the specific response releasing cytokines which both recruit and enhance the activity of other cells, such as the phagocytic macrophages and the NK cells.

The important features to remember about specific immunity are, first, that specific immunity is only induced towards the agent that stimulated it, that is, the immunogen, and, second, that, on second contact with the immunogen, the specific immune response is mobilized more rapidly than on first contact. It is this rapid response which prevents development of the disease in an immune individual because antibodies and cytotoxic cells can attack the microorganism before it causes clinical symptoms. This ability to produce a quicker response on second contact with an immunogen is known as **immunological memory**.

Immunogens

A substance which stimulates a specific immune response is called an immunogen (see *Table 1.6*). Microorganisms and foreign cells, such as foreign red blood cells, are powerful immunogens. This is because they are composed of immunogenic macromolecules such as proteins and glycoproteins. It has been estimated that a protein must have a relative molecular mass (RMM) of at least 5000 Daltons (5 kDa) to be immunogenic and,

Table 1.6 Major groups of immunogens

Immunogen	Example
Microorganisms	Bacteria, viruses, protozoa, multicellular parasites, fungi
Foreign cells	Red blood cells, transplants
Macromolecules	Proteins, glycoproteins, lipoproteins, complex polysaccharides, nucleic acids

generally speaking, the larger the protein, the more immunogenic it will be, so long as it is foreign to the body. Thus, the protein hormone, pig insulin, with a RMM of 5172 Da is weakly immunogenic in humans.

While the term immunogen is used to describe something which stimulates the specific immune response, the term **antigen** is used to describe something which reacts with the products of the immune response. Thus, an antigen may be part of a protein, such as a small polypeptide, which by itself is too small to stimulate specific immunity but, once an immune response has been initiated, is able to combine with the products of that immune response. The word is often used when referring to antibodies reacting with molecules *in vitro*, for example, during an immunoassay such as a radioimmunoassay or in the agglutination tests which are used in the transfusion laboratory.

The word **epitope** is used to describe a region on a protein or glycoprotein immunogen which is recognized by the cells of the specific immune system. It is also that part of the immunogen or antigen to which an antibody can bind. The epitopes on a protein consist of regions of between five and seven amino acids in length, and an immunogenic protein may have a number of epitopes which are recognized as 'foreign' by the cells of the specific immune response. **Haptens** are small molecules which can be rendered immunogenic by attaching them to an immunogenic carrier, rather like adding an extra epitope to a protein (see *Box 1.3*).

Relative importance of humoral and cell-mediated immunity

Most immunogens stimulate both humoral and cell-mediated immunity. However, as a general rule, humoral immunity targets microorganisms that are extracellular parasites, i.e. they live outside the cells of the host. Because antibody is found in the body fluids, including blood and lymph, there is not a problem of access of the antibody to the immunogen. In contrast, CMI is involved with immunity to parasites which live inside cells. Viruses are absolutely dependent on cells for their replication. Certain bacteria, too, habitually live within the cells of the host. Examples of intracellular bacteria include *Mycobacterium tuberculosis*, *Listeria monocytogenes* and *Chlamydia trachomatis*. In this case, antibodies have no access to the parasites and CMI is more significant.

Box 1.3 Haptens

Some relatively small organic molecules, such as dinitrophenol, are too small to stimulate an immune response when administered as the free molecule. However, such small molecules, here known as haptens, can be covalently attached to an immunogenic protein, known as a carrier, to form a hapten–carrier complex. When such complexes are administered to animals by injection, they stimulate the production of antibodies, not only to the protein carrier, but also to the hapten. This implies that the immune system has cells capable of recognizing these small molecules as foreign, but is unable to respond until the haptens are presented to the immune system in the right way (almost as an additional epitope on the carrier protein).

Some drugs, such as penicillin, induce immune haemolytic anaemia when they bind to proteins on red cell membranes and act as haptens, inducing antibody production against them (see Chapter 8).

The ability of the immune system to make antibodies against a range of molecules which are not in themselves immunogenic has been utilized by industry as well as in biological and biomedical research. For example, antibodies against steroid hormones are routinely used to measure the concentration of these hormones in plasma. Antibodies can also be used to detect anabolic steroids and their metabolites in the urine of athletes, and to detect and treat overdoses of digitoxin in patients taking the drug to treat cardiac arrhythmias.

Another application of hapten technology occurs in the production of polysaccharide vaccines. Some bacteria, such as *Haemophilus influenzae* and *Neisseria meningitidis*, both of which can cause meningitis, are covered with a polysaccharide capsule. The polysaccharide is weakly immunogenic and, in a vaccine, induces only a short-term immunity with poor immunological memory. Several vaccines, including those against the bacterial species already mentioned, consist of polysaccharide linked to a protein carrier. These conjugate vaccines induce a more effective immunity with a strong immunological memory.

Specific immune responses are obviously beneficial and they are the chief defences against invasion by microorganisms. There are, however, occasions when immune responses may be inappropriate and even harmful. Humoral immunity, for example, is responsible for a range of allergic reactions including hay fever and allergic asthma. Antibodies are responsible for the blood transfusion reactions, haemolytic anaemias and some occupational diseases such as farmer's lung. CMI is the cause of allergic contact dermatitis and is responsible, at least in part, for the rejection of transplanted tissue. CMI is also responsible for the **graft versus host** reaction, which may be a fatal consequence of stem cell transplantation (see Chapter 12).

1.7 CELLS OF THE SPECIFIC IMMUNE RESPONSE

The cells responsible for the specific immune response are the **small lymphocytes**. Small lymphocytes (see *Fig. 1.1*) are found in the blood, where they comprise approximately 20% of the white blood cells, and in the lymphoid tissues. **Primary lymphoid tissues**, such as the **thymus**, are important sites of maturation for small lymphocytes, whereas the **secondary lymphoid tissues**, such as the spleen, the lymph nodes, the tonsils and mucosa-associated lymphoid tissue (MALT) are the sites of activity of the mature small lymphocytes and are also the places where antibody-producing cells are found.

Development of small lymphocytes

The population of small lymphocytes is one of the most heterogeneous in the body, despite the fact that all small lymphocytes have a very similar appearance. However, it is possible to classify these cells into two major groups, depending initially on where they develop, and into at least three major groups according to their function.

Cells which give rise to small lymphocytes are first produced in the bone marrow, following successive divisions of the **lymphoid stem cells** (see *Fig. 1.2*). During foetal development, some of these immature lymphocytes leave the bone marrow and enter the thymus, a bi-lobed gland found in the upper anterior midline of the chest, where they mature (see *Box 1.4*). Lymphocytes which mature in the thymus are known as **thymus-dependent** or **T lymphocytes**. Two different types of mature T lymphocyte mature in the thymus; these are the **helper T lymphocytes** (T_H) and the **cytotoxic precursor T lymphocytes** (T_C). The function of these cells is discussed below.

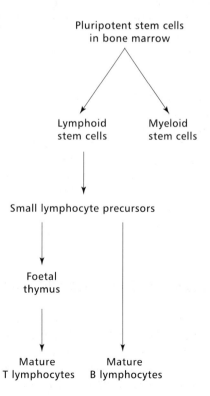

Figure 1.2
Development of small lymphocytes.

In mammals, a second group of small lymphocytes completes its development within the bone marrow. When mature, these cells are known as **B lymphocytes**.

When mature, B and T lymphocytes leave the primary lymphoid tissues and are found in the blood and secondary lymphoid tissues. Small lymphocytes are constantly recirculating between the blood and the lymphoid compartments. They move across the endothelial cells of the blood vessels which supply the lymphoid tissues and enter the lymphatic system. They emerge from lymphoid tissue in the efferent lymph, a fluid which eventually enters the blood supply, at the point where the major lymphatic vessel, the thoracic duct, joins up with the left subclavian vein. Each small lymphocyte responds only to a single epitope and recirculation is essential to ensure that the specific small lymphocytes come into contact with immunogens bearing the epitopes that they recognize.

Box 1.4 The primary lymphoid tissues

The role of the thymus was established in the 1960s when it was shown that removing the thymus from a neonatal mouse (neonatal thymectomy) had profound effects on the immune response. Blood lymphocyte levels were greatly reduced, the spleen and lymph nodes were underdeveloped, CMI was impaired and the animals were very prone to viral infections. Antibody levels were reduced but not absent.

Birds have a second primary lymphoid organ called the Bursa of Fabricius. This organ is not present in mammals. Removing the Bursa of Fabricius from chick embryos was shown to affect humoral immunity but left CMI intact. Bursectomized birds are prone to bacterial, but not viral, infections and antibodies are not found in the plasma. The B lymphocytes were so-called because they are Bursa-dependent in birds. B lymphocytes are responsible for antibody production. In mammals, the 'B' does not stand for bone-marrow derived, because both B and T cells originate in the bone marrow. In fact, B cells in mammals are Bursa equivalent cells because they have the same role in humoral immunity as the Bursa-dependent cells in birds.

Role of T and B lymphocytes

The B lymphocytes are responsible for humoral immunity. When stimulated, they give rise to antibody-producing cells, called **plasma cells** (*Fig. 1.3*). T_C cells, when stimulated, give rise to **cytotoxic T lymphocytes (CTL)**, which are predominantly involved in killing virus-infected cells. T_H are regulatory cells. When stimulated they release an array of cytokines that influence all aspects of the immune response.

Distinguishing T and B lymphocytes

It is not possible to distinguish between T and B lymphocytes or between T_H and T_C in a conventionally stained blood smear. In order to differentiate between them, it is necessary to stain for particular protein markers on the membranes of the individual groups of cells. This can be achieved using

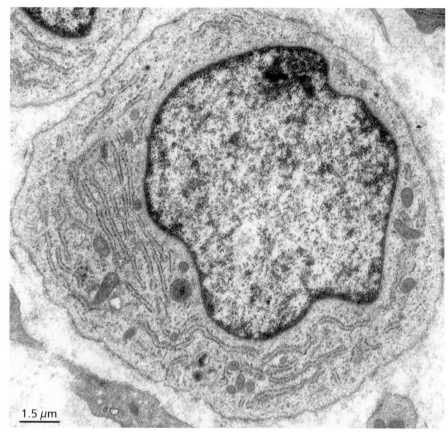

1.5 µm

Figure 1.3
An electron micrograph of a plasma cell (courtesy of Micky Hoult, MMU).

the technique of **immunofluorescence**, using an antibody to the marker in question which has been chemically labelled with a fluorochrome, which is a molecule that emits light when irradiated with light of a shorter wavelength. B lymphocytes have antibodies in their membranes. The cells can be 'stained' with a fluorescent anti-antibody (or anti-immunoglobulin; Chapter 10). All mature T lymphocytes have a membrane-bound molecule known as CD3, which is associated with the T cell receptor and which can be detected with a fluorochrome-labelled anti-CD3. T_H and T_C can be distinguished because the former has the membrane-associated CD4 protein, while the latter has CD8. Thus, use of the appropriate antibody will allow the two cell types to be differentiated.

Specificity of small lymphocytes

All small lymphocytes are specific for a single epitope on an individual immunogen. The specificity of these cells resides in the presence of

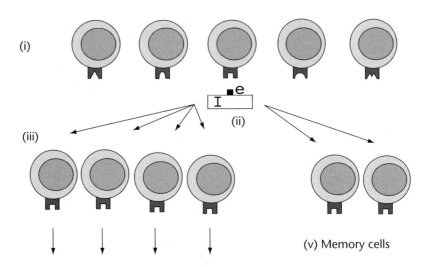

Figure 1.4
Clonal selection: (i) small lymphocytes have receptors for different epitopes; (ii) the
epitope (e) on the immunogen (I) 'selects' the small lymphocyte with the
appropriate receptor. This stimulates proliferation (iii) and differentiation (iv) to
produce effector cells and memory cells (v).

membrane-bound receptors for an individual epitope. The receptors on B
lymphocytes are membrane-bound antibodies, each of which has two
epitope-binding sites. The T cell receptor is composed of two single
polypeptide chains with a single binding site. All the receptors on a single
small lymphocyte, be it a T cell or a B cell, have the same specificity.

When an epitope binds to a receptor on a small lymphocyte, in the appropriate manner, the small lymphocyte starts to proliferate and forms a clone of
identical cells, all with the same specificity (see *Fig. 1.4*), greatly increasing the
number of cells bearing that particular receptor. Most of the cells in this clone
then differentiate, under the influence of a number of cytokines, into '**effector**' cells. Some cells in the clone do not differentiate but remain at this stage
until the next exposure to the same immunogen. These cells are the **memory
cells**. The quicker response shown on second contact with an immunogen is,
at least in part, due to having more of the 'right' sort of cells available.

Activation of B lymphocytes

B lymphocytes have receptors which bind 'native' epitope. This means that
they can be stimulated directly by the epitope as it appears in the immunogen. When B lymphocytes bind the epitope, they proliferate and develop
into plasma cells; that is, fully differentiated antibody-secreting cells (see *Figs
1.3* and *1.5*). Plasma cells do not recirculate but 'home' towards lymphoid
tissues where they continue to secrete antibody until they die, usually within

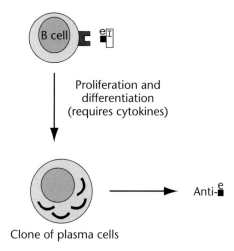

Figure 1.5
Humoral immunity: a B lymphocyte binds to an epitope (e) on an immunogen (I). The cell then proliferates to form a clone of plasma cells, each producing antibody to that epitope. Proliferation and differentiation requires cytokines, supplied by epitope-stimulated helper T lymphocytes.

weeks. The antibody they produce is homogeneous and has the same specificity as the B cell receptor antibodies, ensuring that only the required antibody is produced. In fact, each B cell is only capable of producing antibody of a single specificity and this is determined when the B lymphocyte is developing in the bone marrow. Antibody secreted by plasma cells in lymphoid tissues appears first in the lymph and then in the blood.

Cytokine involvement

The proliferation of B lymphocytes and their differentiation into plasma cells requires cytokines, which are produced by the T_H cells. Certain cytokines favour the production of antibodies of different classes. For example, IL-4 promotes the production of IgE. This requirement for T cells in the production of antibody is seen in the response to most immunogens, which are often referred to as 'T-dependent'. This also explains the poor antibody production in neonatally thymectomized mice.

Polyclonal response

A complex immunogen such as a bacterium or a red blood cell has hundreds of proteins and glycoproteins, each of which has a number of epitopes. Each epitope will stimulate B cells which have receptors for it and, thus, a large number of clones of plasma cells will be produced. These plasma cells secrete antibodies of different specificities because they are responding to many different epitopes. Each antibody will bind to the bacterium or the red blood cell but to different epitopes. For this reason, the normal immune response is said to be **polyclonal**. Antibodies from a single clone of plasma cells are **monoclonal** and are homogeneous (see *Box 1.5*).

Box 1.5 Monoclonal antibodies

Antibodies which are the product of a single clone and which have a single specificity are extremely useful reagents in pathology laboratories. They can, for example, be used in immunoassays, in immuno-fluorescence and flow cytometry, and to identify bacterial or red blood cell antigens (see Chapter 10). Monoclonal antibodies of predetermined specificity are produced by immunizing mice with the relevant immunogen, isolating the plasma cells producing the required antibody and immortalizing the plasma cells by fusing them with mouse myeloma cancer cells. These hybrid myelomas or hybridomas can be grown indefinitely in tissue culture where they continue to produce the same antibody, which can be purified from the culture supernatant. Monoclonal antibodies are invaluable in transfusion science because they represent antibodies of a single specificity and provide a 'reagent' which remains consistent in its qualities. They can be used, for example, in blood grouping, in tissue typing and to purify peripheral blood stem cells for transplantation. It is important to be aware of the difference between polyclonal and monoclonal antibodies and to appreciate that each has advantages and disadvantages depending on the requirements of the laboratory procedure in which they are being used.

Activation of T lymphocytes

Unlike B lymphocytes, T lymphocytes do not respond to antigen in its native state. Instead, they recognize antigen after it has been 'processed' by cells and combined with proteins specified by a region of the genome known as the **major histocompatibility complex (MHC)**. This complex, which is found on chromosome 6 in humans, is discussed in Chapter 12. Genes within this region code for two classes of integral membrane proteins, Class I and Class II MHC proteins. Class I proteins are found on all the nucleated cells in the body whereas Class II proteins are restricted to a few cell types. Both Class I and II MHC proteins are produced in the cytoplasm where they can bind peptides (either self or 'foreign'), and are moved to the membrane where they display the peptide to the relevant cells of the immune system. Each MHC molecule forms a three-dimensional structure in which the bulk of the protein forms a support for a 'peptide-binding groove' into which peptides obtained from proteins can become bound (see *Fig. 1.6*).

Stimulation of T_C cells

The CD8-positive cells which have not yet encountered an immunogen are known as the cytotoxic precursors (T_C) because they give rise, when appropriately stimulated, to the CTL. These cells have the capacity to kill cells infected with a virus for which they are specific. Of course, a T_C does not have access to the interior of a virus-infected cell and the mechanism whereby the T_C recognizes that a cell is infected is intriguing. All nucleated cells in the body are able to display portions of the proteins being produced

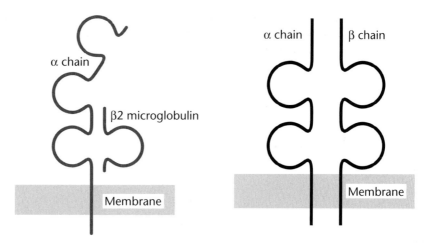

Figure 1.6
MHC Class I (left) and II molecules (courtesy of Micky Hoult, MMU).

inside them, on their membrane. A healthy cell produces many different proteins in its cytoplasm. Within the cytoplasm, small peptides derived from these proteins become bound to the peptide-binding groove of MHC Class I proteins and from here they get transferred to the membrane. It is only in this form that the Tc can recognize the epitope (that is part of the antigen) to which it is specific (see *Fig. 1.7*).

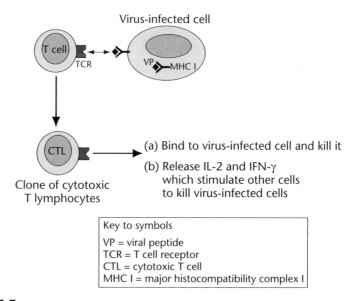

Figure 1.7
Cell-mediated immunity. The T cell receptor on a CD8+ T lymphocyte binds to viral peptide bound to MHC Class I molecules presented on the surface of the infected cell. The T cell is stimulated to proliferate and differentiate into a clone of CTL capable of killing the infected cell directly and indirectly.

Once the T_C has bound to its epitope in the appropriate manner, it is stimulated to divide many times and develops into a clone of CTL. These cells are similar in appearance to T_C, but have a more granular cytoplasm. The granules contain proteins such as **granzymes** and **perforins**, which bring about the destruction of virus-infected cells to which the CTL binds via its specific receptor. Perforins result in the production of pores in the cell membrane while granzymes are endocytosed. They exit from endocytic vesicles through perforin-induced pores and induce self-destruction by stimulating apoptosis.

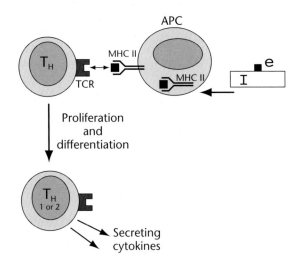

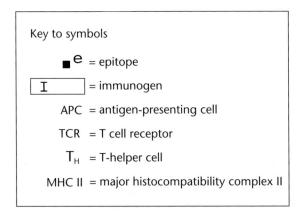

Figure 1.8
Helper T lymphocytes. An immunogen (I) is taken up into an APC and processed within the APC. Peptides from the immunogen are bound to MHC Class II molecules and presented at the surface of the APC. Binding of the T_H to the foreign peptide is followed by proliferation and differentiation into activated, cytokine-secreting T_H.

Stimulation of helper T cells

The role of T_H in all aspects of the immune response cannot be overestimated. When stimulated appropriately by an immunogen, they secrete cytokines, which regulate all aspects of the immune response. Each T_H has epitope-specific receptors which, like the T_C, are unable to recognize native antigen. T_H will only recognize an epitope when the antigen is bound in the peptide-binding groove of an MHC Class II molecule in the membrane of a specialized **antigen-presenting cell (APC)**. Several cell types can act as APC, including monocytes, macrophages, specialized dendritic cells in the blood, interdigitating cells in the lymphoid tissues, and Langerhans cells in the skin. Antigen-presenting cells process foreign or 'exogenous' antigen. This means that they take up the immunogen into membrane-bound endosomes, in which the immunogen is processed by enzymes. Proteins are unfolded and hydrolysed into peptides, which then become bound to MHC Class II molecules (see *Fig. 1.8*). The endosome is then transported along microtubules to the cell periphery where the complex becomes inserted into the cell membrane. The T_H only responds to antigen presented in this form, and must also receive IL-1 secreted by the APC. When stimulated appropriately, the T_H releases cytokines such as IL-2, which stimulates the T_H to divide and to release a whole array of cytokines. Some cytokines are required for the development of humoral immunity and CTL, others stimulate non-

Table 1.7 Cytokine profiles of T_H1 and T_H2 subsets

	T_H1	T_H2
IL-2	+++	---
IFN-γ	+++	---
TNF-β	+++	---
IL-3	+++	+++
GM-CSF*	++	++
IL-4	--	+++
IL-5	--	+++
IL-6	--	++
IL-10	--	+++
IL-12	+++	---
IL-13	---	+++

*Granulocyte-macrophage colony stimulating factor: this is a haemopoeitic factor which promotes the production of polymorphonuclear leucocytes and monocytes by the bone marrow stem cells.

Please note: this is not a complete list of cytokines produced by T_H cells. In addition, it is thought that T_H1 and T_H2 cells are derived from a cell, known as the T_H0 cell, which has a less restricted pattern of cytokine production.

specific cells such as the macrophages (e.g. IFN-γ) and LGL (e.g. IL-2). Some cytokines, e.g. IL-3, are haemopoeitic factors.

There are at least two subsets of T_H cell according to the cytokines that they secrete (see *Table 1.7*). The cytokine profiles produced by T_H1 and T_H2 cells promote the production of cell-mediated and humoral immunity, respectively.

SUGGESTED FURTHER READING

Al-Hasso, S. and Auburn, W.A. Interferons: An Overview. *US Pharmacist* at www.uspharmacist.com. Accessed November 2006.

Baggiolini, M. (2001) Chemokines in pathology and medicine. *Journal of Internal Medicine* **250**, 91–104.

Chatzantoni, K. and Mouzaki, A. (2006) Anti-TNF-α antibody therapies in autoimmune diseases. *Current Topics in Medicinal Chemistry* **6**, 1707–1714.

Delves, P.J., Martin, S., Burton, D. and Roitt, I. (2007) *Roitt's Essential Immunology*, 11th edn. Oxford: Blackwell Publishing.

Goodsell, D.S. (2001) The molecular perspective: interferons. *Oncologist* **6**, 374–375. (An updated version is available at http://www.theoncologist.com/cgi/content/full/6/4/374)

Kindt, T.J., Goldsby, R.A. and Osborne, B.A. (2007) *Kuby Immunology*, 6th edn. London: Freeman.

Muller, W.A. (2003) Leucocyte–endothelial cell interactions in leucocyte transmigration and the inflammatory response. *Trends in Immunology* **24**, 327–364.

Simmons, M.A. (ed.) (2005) *Monoclonal Antibodies: New Research*. Hauppauge, NY: Nova Science Publishers.

Weinstock-Guttman, B. and Jacobs, L.D. (2000) What is new in the treatment of multiple sclerosis? *Drugs* **59**, 401–410.

Wheeler, M.A., Smith, S.D., García-Cardeña, G., Nathan, C.F., Weiss, R.M. and Sessa, W.C. (1997) Bacterial infection induces nitric oxide synthase in human neutrophils. *Journal of Clinical Investigation* **99**, 110–116.

SELF-ASSESSMENT QUESTIONS

1. Why is it incorrect to treat non-specific and specific immune mechanisms as entirely separate entities?
2. List the two major features of specific immunity.
3. Why are interferons regarded as cytokines?
4. Name three 'professional phagocytes' and state where they are found in the body. What is the significance of their location?
5. What is the role of inflammation?
6. When might the acute phase response cause harm?
7. What is the relative importance of humoral immunity and cell-mediated immunity in the defence against infection by microorganisms?

8. Why is a bacterium more immunogenic than a protein?
9. How do B lymphocytes get their name?
10. Why are all small lymphocytes unique prior to antigen stimulation?
11. Why do drugs which inhibit cell division also suppress the immune response?

Antibodies and antigens

Learning objectives
After studying this chapter you should be able to:

■ Describe antibodies as immunoglobulins

■ Classify antibodies into classes and subclasses (where appropriate)

■ Discuss the properties and outline the functions of different antibody classes

■ Describe in detail the structure of IgG

■ Show how the structure of IgG relates to the structures of the other antibody classes

■ Discuss the molecular forces which allow binding between an antibody and an antigen

■ Discuss the significance of antibody affinity and avidity

■ Briefly outline the role of antibodies in causing elimination of an immunogen

■ Appreciate the significance of antibodies in transfusion science

2.1 HISTORY OF ANTIBODIES

Towards the end of the 19th century, evidence had accumulated that when an individual is immunized, the body manufactures specific defence proteins called antibodies which appear in the blood. Indeed, by 1894, the French scientist, Roux, had shown that an antiserum from an immunized horse could cure patients with diphtheria and this form of treatment, known as passive transfer of immunity, was still in use until the use of antibiotics became widespread. In 1900, Landsteiner used 'naturally occurring' antibodies to distinguish the human A, B and O blood group antigens on the surface of human red blood cells (see Chapter 5) and during World War I, tetanus antitoxin, produced in horses, was injected into recently wounded soldiers, to prevent them from getting tetanus.

Despite this long history, the molecular structure of antibodies remained obscure until the Nobel prize winning work of Porter and Edelman in the late

---

Box 2.1 Some useful definitions

In the following chapters, it will be assumed that you are familiar with the following terms:

Plasma: the liquid component of blood separate from the red cells. Plasma contains dissolved proteins including the clotting factors. It can be obtained from blood by adding an anticoagulant to the blood to prevent clotting and centrifuging the blood to remove the cellular component

Serum: the liquid component of the blood after it has been allowed to clot; it therefore does not contain all of the clotting factors (see Chapter 9)

Antiserum: the serum from an animal which has been immunized against an immunogen. It contains antibodies against the immunogen as well as all the other normal components of serum

Antitoxin: an antiserum directed against a toxoid (a toxin which has been chemically treated to render it harmless)

Passive immunization: the process of injecting antibodies in order to treat or prevent an infectious disease

Active immunization: the process of injecting an immunogen in order to stimulate a specific immune response to that immunogen

---

1950s. These days a great deal is known about antibody structure and function. Such things as where antibodies are formed in the body and the complex cellular interactions which allow them to be manufactured are no longer a complete mystery. During the 1970s, even the highly complex genetic mechanisms which allow so many different antibodies to be produced using a comparatively small amount of DNA were beginning to be unravelled. More recently, it has been possible to manufacture monoclonal antibodies produced by immunization of B cells *in vitro* or to engineer genetically 'hybrid' antibodies made from a combination of mouse and human genes, which can be used in treating human cancers. The advance of knowledge in this, as in so many areas of immunology, has been phenomenal. This chapter will examine the biochemical nature of antibodies and how they work.

2.2 ANTIBODIES ARE IMMUNOGLOBULINS

Antibodies are glycoproteins, that is, proteins with a significant amount of carbohydrate attached to them. They are found in all the body fluids including plasma, lymph and secretions such as tears, mucus, saliva and milk. In the blood, they appear mostly in the γ-globulin fraction (see *Fig. 2.1*), although they extend into the β- and α-globulin regions. Antibodies are such a heterogeneous group of molecules that they are known collectively as **immunoglobulins**, that is, globulins with an immune function. This name was coined by international agreement in 1964, at the same time as they were classified according to their different properties.

Immunoglobulins are classified into five **classes** or **isotypes**. Individuals have antibodies of all five classes in their blood. Antibody classes were first defined by their antigenicity, which means that antibodies raised against one class of immunoglobulin reacted only with that class and no other. The five

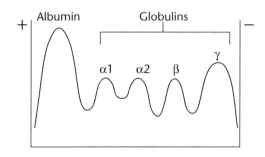

Figure 2.1
Electrophoresis of plasma. When plasma is subjected to electrophoresis on cellulose acetate at pH 8.6, it separates into several fractions, depending on the charge of the proteins at that pH. Most antibodies are found within the γ-globulin faction, which is the slowest moving fraction.

classes of antibody are all prefixed with **Ig**, standing for immunoglobulin: IgM, IgG, IgA, IgD and IgE. These antibodies differ with respect to their structure, physicochemical properties, their distribution and concentrations as well as their functions. Some properties of these different classes are shown in *Table 2.1*.

Table 2.1   Properties of different antibody classes

Class	Mean serum concentration (mg ml^{-1})	Relative molecular mass (Da)	Carbohydrate (as %)
IgM	1.5	900 000	12
IgG	13.5	150 000	2–3
IgA	3.5	160 000–385 000	7–11
IgD	0.03	184 000	9–14
IgE	0.00005	188 000	12

Within some antibody classes, there are also subclasses. Again, these were originally defined by their antigenicity, i.e. while an antiserum raised against the class will react with all the subclasses, there are some antisera which will only react with a particular subclass. These differences in antigenicity reflect basic differences in the amino acid sequences between the subclasses. Humans have four subclasses of IgG and two subclasses of IgA.

2.3   KINETICS OF THE ANTIBODY RESPONSE

Before looking at the structure and function of the different antibody classes, it is necessary to consider the differences between the antibody

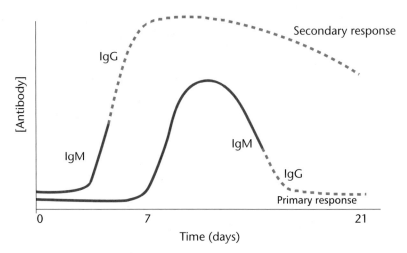

Figure 2.2
Kinetics of the antibody response. The primary and secondary antibody responses differ in several ways: the length of the latent period (i.e. before antibody can be detected), the total amount of antibody, the duration of the response, the predominant class of antibody and the antibody affinity. (Courtesy of Micky Hoult, MMU.)

responses in a non-immune and an immune animal. In order to illustrate this, consider an experimental situation in which an animal, such as a rabbit, is immunized with an immunogen, such as bovine serum albumin (BSA). The animal is immunized with BSA by injection on day 0 (see *Fig. 2.2*). Samples of blood are taken at daily intervals and the serum tested for the presence of antibodies to the BSA. In an animal which has never been previously immunized with BSA, there is a delay period of approximately 7 days before any anti-BSA can be detected. This delay is known as the **latent period**. After this, antibody levels rise steadily, reach a peak and then fall to pre-immunization levels by around 21 days. This response, in a non-immune animal, is known as the **primary response**. Most of the antibody produced in a primary response belongs to the IgM class, while IgG is only detected towards the end of the response.

When an animal which is immune to BSA – that is, has already gone through a primary response – is re-injected with BSA, a completely different sort of response, **the secondary response**, is seen. There is a shorter latent period, the antibody concentration is higher and the response lasts for much longer (typically weeks or even months). Although IgM is detected at the start of the response, the predominant antibody is IgG. In addition, the antibody produced in a secondary response binds much more strongly to the immunogen reflecting the production of antibodies with higher **affinity** for the immunogen. This is analogous to the response which occurs in a patient when transfused with blood containing foreign blood group antigens. The second occasion of transfusion with the foreign antigens results in a rapid and stronger immune response.

The response in animals to injection of human proteins has been used in the production of 'anti-human globulin', the antibody used in the antiglobulin test described in Chapter 10.

Knowledge of the kinetics of the antibody response is useful when assessing the immune status of an individual. For example, all pregnant women in the UK are tested for antibodies to rubella (German measles). If they have IgM antibodies, it probably indicates a recent infection, which might have clinical consequences for the baby. Knowledge of the kinetics of an immune response is also useful when raising antibodies for use, e.g. in clinical studies. If IgG is required, as is most often the case, the antiserum is only taken after a series of immunizations.

2.4 IMMUNOGLOBULIN ISOTYPES

IgM (the M is derived from its original name, β_2 (or γ_1)-**macroglobulin**) is always the first antibody to be produced in an immune response and is the predominant antibody of the primary response. Elevated levels of IgM, therefore, usually indicate recent infection. IgM makes up approximately 10% of the immunoglobulins in plasma. The majority of IgM is found in the blood, relatively little being found in lymph and negligible amounts in secretions, though traces may be found in milk. IgM is a very effective antibacterial antibody for several reasons, not least is its ability to activate complement. The 'naturally occurring' antibodies to the antigens of the ABO blood groups are almost always IgM antibodies. They do not, therefore, pose any threat to an ABO-incompatible foetus because IgM antibodies do not cross the placenta. However, they are of considerable consequence in the case of ABO-incompatible transfusions (see Chapters 5 and 11, and *Box 2.2*).

Box 2.2 Natural antibodies

The antibodies of the ABO system are often called 'naturally occurring antibodies' because they are present apparently without immunization with the appropriate red cells. Children have only low levels of these antibodies, indicating that they are produced, as expected, in response to exposure to immunogens. In fact, bacteria also possess antigens of the same type as the A and B antigens and people produce antibodies against these bacterial antigens which they themselves do not have on their red cells (see Chapter 5). The fact that these antibodies are usually of the IgM class also indicates that they are produced in response to bacterial carbohydrate antigens.

Immunoglobulin G (IgG) is the most abundant antibody in blood and makes up approximately 75% of the immunoglobulins in the plasma. IgG is found in both the vascular and extravascular compartments and is evenly distributed between the two (45% and 55%, respectively). It is the predominant antibody of the secondary response. In addition, IgG is the only antibody which crosses the placenta and therefore protects the developing foetus against infections. Newborn babies have adult levels of IgG in their blood but this is almost entirely of maternal origin. This antibody is catabolized fairly quickly so that, by between 3 and 6 months of age, babies have only low IgG levels. Thereafter, the levels begin to rise steadily, as the infant is exposed to environmental immunogens (and vaccinations) and starts to produce its own IgG. The fact that IgG crosses the placenta has implications for a foetus if the mother is immunized against foetal red blood cell antigens. This can happen, for example, in an (Rh)-negative mother who has developed antibodies to Rh antigens on the red cells of an Rh-positive foetus (see Chapters 6 and 8). The passage of anti-red cell antibodies across the placenta may lead to the development of haemolytic disease of the newborn.

IgG exists in four **subclasses** (or sub-isotypes) in man (IgG_{1-4}), the most abundant of which is IgG_1. IgG_3 has a larger relative molecular mass (RMM) but the distribution of the different classes between the vascular and extravascular compartments and the extent of glycosylation is very similar. These subclasses have complementary roles in the immune response. With the exception of IgG_3, IgG has the longest half-life of the immunoglobulin classes and this persistence makes it suitable for passive immunization, e.g. for treatment of active infection or as a treatment for the prevention of Rh isoimmunization. The ability of an antibody to affect a transfused patient clinically is dependent upon the IgG subclass.

Immunoglobulin A (IgA) is found in plasma, extravascular fluid and secretions. It exists in different forms depending on where it is located. In humans, most IgA in the serum exists as a 160 000 Da molecule, though a proportion occurs as a dimer of this structure. The vast majority of IgA is found in the secretions and this form is larger. In addition, two subclasses of IgA are found: IgA_1 and IgA_2, the former being the most abundant (3.0 mg ml^{-1} plasma and 0.5 mg ml^{-1} plasma, respectively). The two subclasses have similar distributions, and half-lives of approximately 6 days.

While it is not known whether plasma IgA has any particular function, secretory IgA is known to protect the mucosal surfaces from infections. This is a significant function because the total area of mucosal membranes in humans has been estimated at 400 m^2, the largest area of 'exposed' surface in the body. Far more IgA is made at these sites in total even than IgG, which is secreted into the lymph. Organisms which routinely enter the body via the gut, for example, may be prevented from doing so by the presence of plasma cells in the gut actively secreting IgA. It is therefore more effective to immunize against these pathogens by local immunization, e.g. oral vaccines against poliomyelitis, though this must be balanced by any risk of the virus reverting to a more virulent form by this route. IgA is known to be more efficient in the presence of the anti-bacterial enzyme lysozyme, although the mechanism of this interaction is uncertain. Around 1 in 700 caucasians have a deficiency of IgA. This has implications in transfusion as they often react to the IgA in transfused blood by forming anti-IgA antibodies (see Chapter 9).

Immunoglobulin E (IgE) is found in low concentrations in plasma and has the shortest half-life at a mere 2 days. The low concentrations of free

IgE can be explained partly by the fact that IgE has the ability to bind to a receptor on the surface of basophils in the blood and mast cells in the tissues. This receptor is of high affinity so will bind IgE even when the latter is present at such low concentrations. The binding of IgE to these receptors indicates its role in stimulating inflammation (see below) and reflects its importance in helping to eliminate multicellular parasites such as nematodes (roundworms) and helminths from the body. In addition, when produced in response to a 'harmless' immunogen, such as grass pollen, in genetically susceptible individuals, IgE can cause the symptoms of allergy, including hay fever, allergic asthma and food allergies.

Immunoglobulin D (IgD) is not considered to have any role as a soluble antibody, though it does occur as a receptor on B lymphocytes. IgD is found in relatively low concentrations in plasma where it probably represents IgD receptors which have been shed from the surface of B lymphocytes. All antibody classes can be found as receptors on B lymphocytes and sometimes a cell will display more than one class of receptor. IgD, for example, is frequently found together with IgM.

2.5 ANTIBODY STRUCTURE

IgG was the first class of antibody to have its structure determined. The work of the British scientist, Rodney Porter, and the American, Gerald Edelman, was paramount in this investigation, a fact recognized by the shared award of a Nobel prize for medicine in 1972. Porter studied the fragments produced when the proteolytic enzymes pepsin and papain were incubated with purified rabbit IgG for limited amounts of time. Edelman studied the effects of mercaptoethanol, which reduces disulphide bonds, on the antibody. When a protein consists of several polypeptide chains held together by disulphide links, mercaptoethanol will reduce these links and cause the chains to fall apart (see *Box 2.3*).

The results of these investigations led to the proposal for the structure of IgG which is still held today.

Box 2.3 Investigating the structure of IgG

When Porter incubated IgG with papain for a limited time, and separated the fragments by ion exchange chromatography, he found that some fragments could still bind a single molecule of antigen. These he called Fab (fragment antigen-binding). The other fragments did not bind antigen but could be crystallized out and he called these Fc (fragment crystallizable). There were twice as many Fab fragments as Fc. When he digested IgG with pepsin, he obtained a single large fragment which could bind two molecules of hapten and which he called the Fab'$_2$ fragment.

When Edelman treated IgG with mercaptoethanol and separated the chains by gel filtration, he obtained two sorts of chain, one half the size of the other. Their RMMs indicated that each IgG had two of the 'heavy' chains and two of the 'light' chains. Take a look at *Fig. 2.3*. Try to predict what will happen if the molecule is broken to the left or the right of the disulphide link between the heavy chains. Now predict where papain and pepsin digest the molecule.

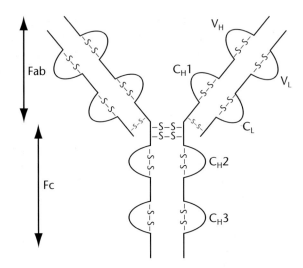

Figure 2.3
The structure of an IgG molecule. The molecule consists of heavy (H) and light (L) chains as shown, held together by disulphide links to form two Fab and one Fc regions. V and C refer to variable and constant regions, as described in the text. Each V region consists of a single domain (V_H, V_L), while the constant region has three domains (C_H1, C_H2 and C_H3).

A single molecule of IgG consists of four polypeptide chains held together by disulphide links (see *Fig. 2.3*). Two of these chains have a RMM of 25 000 Da and are called the light (L) chains. The two light chains in an individual antibody molecule are identical. The other two chains, the heavy (H) chains, have a RMM of 50 000 Da and are also identical to each other. The heavy chains of all IgG molecules have certain similarities in terms of amino acid sequences and are known as γ chains. These are different from the heavy chains of the other classes of antibody. In fact, the classification of antibodies is based on similarities in heavy chain structure within a particular class (see *Table 2.2*). It is for this reason that antisera raised against IgG heavy chains will not react with IgM heavy chains and *vice versa*.

Table 2.2 The immunoglobulin heavy chains

Antibody class	Type of heavy chain
IgG	γ
IgM	μ
IgA	α
IgE	ε
IgD	δ

The heavy and light chains of IgG are joined together in such a way as to produce a symmetrical molecule with two identical regions known as Fab (fragment antigen-binding) regions and a single Fc (fragment crystallizable) region. Each Fab region is composed of the light chain and part of the heavy chain. Because an individual IgG molecule has two binding sites, it is said to be divalent.

While, by definition, all IgG molecules have γ heavy chains, the situation is somewhat different with light chains. Only two different forms of light chain exist and these have been designated kappa (κ) light chains and lamda (λ) light chains. They differ in amino acid sequence (all κ chains having certain similarities to other κ light chains and similarly for λ light chains). These light chains may be associated with any of the heavy chain types with the proviso that both the light chains in an individual antibody molecule are always of the same type. Thus, an antibody belongs to the IgG class whether it contains two κ chains and two γ chains or two λ chains and two γ chains.

Immunoglobulin domains

In addition to the interchain disulphide bonds which join the chains together, there are also intrachain disulphide bonds formed between cysteine residues that are separated by approximately 60 amino acids. Such bonding has the effect of forming a loop in the chain. There are four such loops in the γ chain and two in each of the light chains. Each loop occurs within a region known as a **domain**, which contains 100–110 amino acids and a single disulphide loop. All immunoglobulins, as well as several other molecules in the immune system, have a similar domain-type structure. Within the domain, there is a similar pattern of folding of the polypeptide chain.

The molecules which have this immunoglobulin 'domain' structure are thought to have evolved from the same primitive ancestral gene and are thus related in evolutionary terms. The molecules are often referred to as the **immunoglobulin superfamily**. They include the T cell receptor, the CD4 and CD8 molecules on T lymphocytes and the MHC Class I and II molecules which are so important in antigen presentation (see Chapter 1).

Role of the Fab and Fc regions

The roles of the Fab and Fc regions of an antibody molecule reflect the two main roles of that antibody. These are, first, to bind specifically to the epitope and, second, to stimulate the elimination of the immunogen, the latter being stimulated by the former.

It is the Fab region which binds to the epitope, while the Fc region is responsible for mediating the other effector role(s) of the antibody such as activating complement and binding to phagocytic cells. All antibodies are specific for an individual epitope and, for this reason, all antibodies produced by different clones of plasma cells against different epitopes must have different structures. On the other hand, there are relatively few ways in which antibodies can stimulate the elimination of an immunogen, so, in this respect, all antibodies of the same class must be similar in structure.

The paradox that all antibodies are different but all antibodies are the same was neatly confirmed in experiments in which the heavy chains and light chains of many different IgG molecules were analysed for their primary structure, i.e. the sequence of amino acids which makes up the polypeptide structure. Analysis of a number of different γ chains revealed that the sequence of amino acids in one section of the heavy chain was very similar in all the chains studied. This sequence constitutes 75% of the γ chain at the C-terminal end of the molecule (approximately 330 amino acids) and is known as the **constant**, or **C**-region. It is made up of three domains as shown in *Fig. 2.3*. However, the remaining 25% of the chain, starting at the N-terminal end and comprising a single domain, had an amino acid sequence which differed in all the γ chains studied. This domain is known as the **variable**, or **V**-region.

A similar result was found when a number of different κ chains (or λ chains) were sequenced. In this case, the constant region and variable regions occupy approximately half the light chain at the C-terminal and N-terminal ends. Thus, the variability occurs at the Fab end of the molecule. In fact, the antigen-binding site is made up of the variable region of a light chain and a heavy chain. The sequence in each variable region is unique for each antibody which is the product of a different plasma cell. It is this unique sequence which determines the specificity of the antibody. The least variable part of the antibody corresponds to the Fc region, which mediates the other biological functions of the antibody.

Hypervariable regions

When the sequences of a number of variable regions on κ, λ or γ chains were analysed in more depth, it was discovered that there were different degrees of variability even within the variable regions. For example, sequences of a number of variable regions of γ chains revealed that some parts of these regions were even more variable than the rest. There were three such hypervariable regions for every V region studied (whether light or heavy) and these are very important structures for determining the specificity of the antibody. They are nowadays referred to as the **complementarity determining regions (CDR)** and the six CDR in each Fab region (three from the heavy and three from the light chain) give the binding site a unique 'shape' into which only the epitope will fit well. The 'less variable' regions between and around the CDR are called the '**framework**' regions, and they support the CDR which form the shape of the binding site.

Structure of IgM

As was previously mentioned, the heavy chains of IgM are larger than those of IgG and this is because they have an extra domain in the constant region,

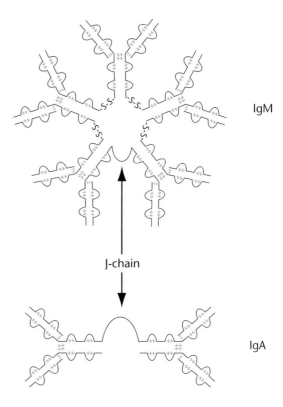

Figure 2.4
The structure of IgM and IgA. IgM is a
pentamer made up of five four-chain 'units'
linked by a J-chain and by disulphide bonds.
IgA may take the form of a dimer linked by a
J-chain.

i.e. they have one variable and four constant domains). However, the increase
in the size of the heavy chains alone cannot account for the RMM of 900 000
Da. The difference between them lies in the fact that IgM is polymeric, where
the monomeric unit is the basic four-chain structure as already discussed
with reference to IgG. IgM is actually a pentamer, containing five of these
four chain units (see *Fig. 2.4*). The five units are joined together through
disulphide links between the Fc regions and through an additional protein,
the J-chain (RMM 15 000 Da), which links two of the four-chain structures.
The J-chain is produced within the plasma cell and assembled along with the
heavy and light chains. Theoretically, a pentameric IgM having ten Fab sites
should be able to bind ten molecules of the epitope. In practice, the number
bound is nearer to five, and this seems to be due to constraints of size: there
is not enough room to 'fit' ten epitopes around the molecule.

Immunoglobulins A, E and D

The majority of plasma IgA of humans is present in a monomeric form.
However, IgA can also exist as a dimer, which is held together through disulphide bonds and a J-chain (see *Fig. 2.4*) Secretory IgA also occurs as a dimer,
held together by a J-chain, and with an additional protein, the **secretory
component**, wrapped around the joined Fc regions of the dimer. The secretory component (RMM 70 000 Da) is produced by epithelial cells through
which IgA passes as it is secreted. The secretory component probably serves
to protect the antibody from the action of proteolytic enzymes in hostile

environments such as the gut. It is also possible that this component actually facilitates secretion.

IgE has a monomeric form. Its large RMM (188 000 Da) reflects the larger heavy chains which, like the μ chains of IgM, have an additional constant region domain. IgE molecules are also quite heavily glycosylated, though the precise role of the carbohydrate is not certain.

IgD is found in very low concentrations in the plasma, though it is more abundant as a membrane-associated B-cell receptor. Its relatively RMM is not due to extra domains but to an extended hinge region. This antibody has a short half-life owing to an extreme susceptibility to enzymic proteolysis.

2.6 BINDING OF AN ANTIBODY TO AN EPITOPE

At this point, a little revision might be useful. Remember that an epitope is a small region of an immunogen to which an antibody binds. It may be a short sequence of a protein (about five to seven amino acids in size), for example the short peptide loops on the surface of cells possessing the RhD antigen, or an oligosaccharide forming part of a glycoprotein or glycolipid, for example the antigens of the ABO system (see Chapter 5) or it may be a hapten, a molecule which has been deliberately attached to a protein in order to stimulate antibody production. In essence, the epitope is relatively small compared with the whole antibody molecule but not necessarily when compared with the antibody-binding site. Remember, too, that the term antigen is given to a molecule which combines with an antibody, and is often used when discussing reactions occurring *in vitro*. Both terms will be used in this chapter.

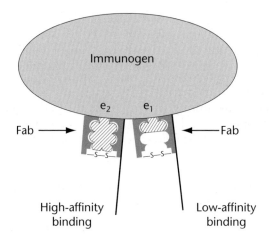

Figure 2.5
Binding of antibody to an epitope. When the Fab site is complementary in shape to the epitope, high-affinity binding can occur. Alternatively, an epitope may fit less well into the binding site, to give low-affinity binding.

The interaction between an antibody and an epitope has been likened to a 'lock and key' mechanism, where the epitope is the 'key' and the binding site is the 'lock'. Essentially, the prime consideration as to whether an antibody will bind an epitope is the complementarity between the shape of the binding site and the shape of the epitope (see *Fig. 2.5*). When they are complementary, the epitope will fit well into the binding site, allowing amino acid residues in the antibody to fit close to residues making up the epitope, and allowing secondary interactions to take place which stabilize the binding. These other forces are described in *Table 2.3* and Chapter 10. Note that there are no covalent interactions between the antibody and the epitope. The reaction is reversible and is governed by the law of mass action. However, if there is good fit between the antibody and the epitope, there will be high-affinity binding and separating the two molecules will be difficult to achieve.

Table 2.3   Forces holding the antibody/antigen together

Force	Origin
Hydrophobic interactions	Between molecules which come together because they mutually expel water
Hydrogen bonds	Where hydrogen is shared between electronegative atoms such as nitrogen and oxygen
Electrostatic interaction	Between oppositely charged groups
Van der Waal's forces	Interactions between electron clouds around molecules

Antibody affinity and avidity

The binding of an antibody-binding site to the epitope is a chemical reaction and can be defined by certain characteristics. One of the most useful is the term **affinity**. This is a precise chemical description which is a measure of the strength of binding of a single antibody binding site to a univalent hapten (that is, one with only one epitope). The affinity of an antibody is an important property and it governs, for example, whether or not this antibody will be useful *in vitro* for the detection of blood group antigens. *In vivo*, the antibody affinity will influence the pathological consequences of unwanted antibodies, such as antibodies to red blood cells in haemolytic anaemia.

Consider the following reaction: antibody + antigen $\rightleftharpoons$ immune complex or:

$$Ab + Ag \rightleftharpoons AbAg$$

According to the law of mass action, the rate of the forward reaction is proportional to the concentration of the reactants or:

$$r_1 \, \alpha \, [Ab] \times [Ag]$$

or

$$r_1 = k_1 \, [Ab] \times [Ag]$$

where k_1 is the rate constant for the forward reaction.

Conversely, the rate of the backward reaction (r_2) is proportional to the concentration of the product or:

$$r_2 = k_2 \, [AbAg]$$

At equilibrium, the rates of the forward and backward reactions are balanced and $r_1 = r_2$; therefore:

$$k_1 \, [Ab] \times [Ag] = k_2 \, [AbAg]$$

and

$$k_1/k_2 = [AbAg]/[Ab] \times [Ag]$$

The figure k_1/k_2 is the **association constant, K**, or **affinity**, and its units are $l \, mol^{-1}$ when the concentrations of the reactants are given in $l \, mol^{-1}$. An antibody with an association constant of $10^5 \, l \, mol^{-1}$ does not bind as strongly as an antibody with an affinity of $10^7 \, l \, mol^{-1}$.

Sometimes the term affinity is expressed as the reciprocal of K. This has units of concentration and is in many ways easier to understand. For example, a figure of $1/K$ of $10^{-8} \, l \, mol^{-1}$ would indicate a concentration of the hapten required in order to ensure that half the antibody-binding sites were occupied. In this case, the lower the concentration of antigen required to achieve 50% binding, the higher the affinity.

The affinity, as defined above, refers to the binding of a homogeneous antibody to a single epitope or a univalent antigen, such as a hapten. Apart from monoclonal antibodies, antibodies produced in animals are very heterogeneous, because they are the product of a polyclonal response. The affinity which is actually measured in such a preparation is the average of the affinities of all the antibodies in that preparation and K is the **average association constant**.

Most immunogens have many different epitopes. An antiserum prepared against such an immunogen will contain antibodies against many epitopes and there will be a range of antibodies of different affinities against all these different epitopes. Measuring the strength of binding of an antiserum against a multivalent antigen is therefore less precise than measuring the reaction between the binding of a single antibody to a single epitope. The term **avidity** is used to denote the strength of binding between antibodies and multivalent antigens or immunogens. In addition, the number of Fab sites on the antibody is also important in determining the strength of binding. For example, IgM will bind to an immunogen containing a repeated epitope with higher avidity simply because it has ten binding sites, even if the affinity of each binding site is relatively low.

2.7 EFFECTOR ROLE OF THE ANTIBODY

The secondary role of the antibody is stimulated following binding to the immunogen. Various activities may be stimulated following binding and these are summarized in *Table 2.4*.

Table 2.4 Effector activities of antibodies

Activity	Antibody classes involved
Bring about physical changes to the immunogen, e.g. agglutination of cells and precipitation of proteins	IgM, IgG, IgA
Trigger lysis of cellular immunogens through activation of complement	IgM, IgG
Trigger inflammation	IgM, IgG, IgE
Increase the efficiency of uptake and destruction by phagocytic cells	IgM, IgG, IgA
Trigger lysis of cellular immunogens through antibody-dependent cellular cytotoxicity	IgG

The importance of each of these activities depends to a certain extent on the location of the antigen/antibody reaction, on the nature of the immunogen and on the class of antibody involved.

Physical changes

An antibody binding to a soluble immunogen, such as a toxin, can precipitate the protein out of solution. This happens if antibody and antigen are present in the proportions needed to produce a large lattice-like complex of antibodies and antigens. Precipitation depends upon the antigen being multivalent, i.e. having several epitopes and sufficient antibody to produce the 'optimal proportions' required. *In vivo*, this may serve the purpose of making the complex more easily phagocytosed. Only those antibodies normally present in sufficient concentration may be regarded as precipitating, i.e. IgM, IgG and IgA (see *Fig. 2.6*).

When an antibody is directed against a cell rather than a soluble protein, the combination may cause the cells to clump together or **agglutinate**. IgM is the most efficient agglutinating antibody. Indeed, IgG is unable to agglutinate red cells directly owing to the negative surface charge of these cells and this will be discussed in some detail in Chapter 10.

The physical changes brought about when an antibody combines with an antigen can be used in tests to detect either antigen or antibody (see *Box 2.4* and Chapter 10).

Lysis

Antibodies may cause lysis of cellular immunogens in two different ways. First, antibodies of the IgG and IgM classes activate complement. In effect, antibodies binding to the membranes of cells activate a series of reactions which result in lysis. IgM is the most efficient lytic antibody, but IgG can also activate complement. In blood transfusion reactions, much of the

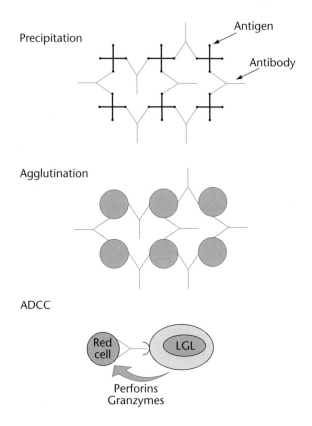

Figure 2.6
Secondary role of the antibody. An antibody may precipitate soluble proteins (top) or agglutinate cells (middle) by forming multiple crosslinks between the molecules of antigen and antibody. IgG may lyse cells (bottom) by binding via the Fc region to large granular lymphocytes (LGL), stimulating the latter to release perforins and granzymes.

pathology involves the activation of complement. This topic is discussed in some detail in Chapter 3.

Antibodies also cause lysis of cells by triggering the activity of large granular lymphocytes (LGL). LGL have membrane-bound receptors for the Fc region of IgG (FcγR). Thus, when an IgG molecule binds to a cell via its Fab region, the Fc region will bind to the LGL. When this happens, the LGL is triggered to release proteins in its granular cytoplasm which destroy the membrane of the target cell (see *Fig. 2.6*). This type of killing is known as **antibody-dependent cellular cytotoxicity (ADCC)** and is only mediated by IgG. The process is very efficient in terms of the amount of antibody required, which is, in theory, a single antibody molecule per target cell. ADCC can also be carried out by monocytes and has been used to test for the clinical significance of anti-Rh antibodies.

Antibodies which bring about the lysis of red cells are called **haemolysins**.

(Note that cells of the placenta also possess the receptor FcγR, which is responsible for the transfer of IgG antibodies into the foetus).

Box 2.4 Precipitation and agglutination tests

Assays and tests which are based on the precipitation of an antigen by antibody are used in pathology laboratories worldwide. For example, nephelometry is a rapid and sensitive method used to quantify plasma proteins. It relies on the properties of immunoprecipitates formed in a cuvette to scatter light passed through the mixture of antibody and antigen. Radial immunodiffusion (RID) and rocket electrophoresis are also used to quantify proteins, but in both methods the precipitate is allowed to form in an agar or agarose gel. With RID, the antibody is incorporated evenly into the agar while the antigen is introduced into wells cut into the agar. As the antigen diffuses out of the well, a circle of precipitation is formed (see *Fig. 2.7*), the square of the diameter being proportional to the antigen concentration. Rocket electrophoresis is similar in principle, but in this case the antigen is electrophoresed into the agar, forming precipitation 'rockets', the area of which is related to the antigen concentration.

Agglutination tests are used in microbiology as well as in the transfusion science laboratory. IgG and IgM can effectively agglutinate bacteria and, even today, a number of laboratory tests to determine immune status to a microorganism are based on agglutination. Antibodies are very discriminatory and have allowed the classification of bacteria into species, groups, subgroups and strains. Agglutination tests are the most common test used in transfusion science for determining blood groups and antibodies that bring about agglutination of red cells are called haemagglutinins. They are discussed in Chapter 10.

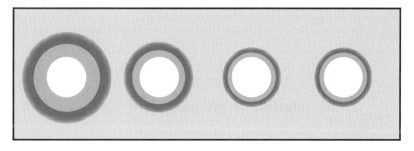

Figure 2.7
Single radial immunodiffusion (SRID). Antibody is incorporated evenly into an agar or agarose gel (1–2% agar in saline). Wells are punched into the agar and equal volumes of antigen solution at different concentrations are added to the wells. As antigen diffuses radially, a circular precipitate is produced around the well. When all the antigen has diffused the square of the diameter is directly proportional to the antigen concentration. (Courtesy of Micky Hoult, MMU.)

Stimulation of inflammation

The binding of antibodies to an antigen may stimulate inflammation in several ways. For example, when complement is activated by IgG or IgM bound to an antigen, a number of pharmacologically active proteins are produced (see Chapter 3). Some of these components have **anaphylatoxin** activity. This means that they bind to mast cells in the tissues and basophils in the blood and stimulate them to degranulate. The histamine released from these cells triggers inflammation. The inflammatory process serves to allow plasma containing complement and antibodies to enter an inflammatory site and may also result in the exudation of neutrophils into the inflamed area, thus promoting phagocytosis.

IgE is a potent activator of inflammation. Mast cells and basophils have high-affinity receptors for the Fc region of IgE (FcεRI). Much of the IgE that is produced in the body becomes bound to these receptors. Degranulation of mast cells and basophils is triggered when an antigen crosslinks two specific IgE molecules on the surface of these cells. The histamine released triggers inflammation. Other pharmacologically active agents are also released which, together with histamine, cause a variety of effects including smooth muscle contraction, increased mucus secretion and the accumulation of eosinophils at the site of release (see *Box 2.5*).

Box 2.5 IgE and the elimination of multicellular parasites

The potent effect of IgE in triggering inflammation reflects its role *in vivo*, which is to eliminate multicellular parasites such as tapeworms and nematodes. Multicellular worms cannot be lysed by complement and are much too large to be engulfed by phagocytes. Worm antigens crosslink worm-specific IgE on the surface of mast cells, for example, in the gut. The subsequent response, including inflammation, histamine-induced contraction of smooth muscle in the gut and increased mucus production, helps to expel the worm. Unfortunately, in genetically susceptible people, IgE may also be produced in response to inappropriate antigens such as pollen, animal dandruff or dander, and the faeces of house dust mites. This leads to the development of hay fever and allergic asthma.

Stimulation of phagocytosis

The binding of antibodies to an antigen may stimulate phagocytosis in several ways. For example, there are antibody receptors on phagocytic cells. An antibody bound to an antigen may subsequently bind to a phagocyte through these receptors. This has the effect not just of bringing the antigen and the phagocyte together, but also of amplifying many of the activities of the phagocyte including uptake of antigen, the respiratory burst and the production of hypochlorite, all of which are involved in killing phagocytosed microorganisms.

Receptors for the Fc region of IgG are widely distributed on phagocytic cells. Three different types of FcγR are now recognized. In addition, phagocytic cells may also have receptors for the Fc regions of other antibodies such as IgA.

Antibodies also stimulate phagocytosis in several ways through the activation of complement. For example, some activated complement proteins are chemotactic factors for neutrophils. Phagocytic cells also have receptors for a variety of complement proteins, including products of activation of C3. Thus, complement can also opsonize antigens and stimulate uptake by phagocytes. Red blood cells also have C3 receptors, enabling them to pick up immune complexes and transport them to the spleen and liver, where the complexes are stripped from their surfaces and phagocytosed by macrophages. This is a significant mechanism for removal of complexes owing to the sheer numbers of red cells in the blood. Phagocytic neutrophils and complement play an important role in the removal of 'damaged' red cells from the circulation, for example red cells which have antibodies bound to their surface. This process results in the anaemia seen in immune and autoimmune haemolytic anaemia (see Chapter 8). Most IgG antibodies to red blood cells cause red cell destruction extravascularly by the interaction of the Fc region of IgG with Fcγ receptors on mononuclear cells such as monocytes.

SUGGESTED FURTHER READING

Delves, P.J., Martin, S., Burton, D. and Roitt, I. (2007) *Roitt's Essential Immunology*, 11th edn. Oxford: Blackwell Publishing.

Kindt, T.J., Goldsby, R.A. and Osborne, B.A. (2007) *Kuby Immunology*, 6th edn. London: Freeman.

Price, C.P. and Newman, D.J. (2001) *Principles and Practice of Immunoassay*. London: Macmillan.

Todd, I. and Spickett, G. (2005) *Lecture Notes on Immunology*, 5th edn. Oxford: Blackwell Science.

SELF-ASSESSMENT QUESTIONS

1. Which of the immunoglobulins is: (a) the most abundant in blood; (b) always produced first in an immune response; (c) involved in the elimination of parasites; (d) the most abundant in secretions?
2. What is the basis for classifying the immunoglobulins?
3. Why is IgG used for passive immunization?
4. State two ways in which the structure of IgM differs from that of IgG.
5. Distinguish between the constant and variable regions of heavy chains.
6. Name two roles of the Fc region of IgG.
7. List three forces involved in the binding of an antibody to an antigen.
8. Distinguish between the terms **affinity** and **avidity**.
9. Name two ways in which IgG can promote phagocytosis.

Complement

3.1 HISTORICAL CONTEXT

Towards the end of the 19th century, several scientists recorded the presence of a heat-labile substance in fresh serum which was able to **complement** the activity of antibodies. For example, Buchner in 1893 reported the loss of bactericidal activity in a serum after it had been heated to 56°C. In 1895, Bordet, to whom the discovery of complement is often attributed, showed that the ability of an antiserum to kill the bacteria which cause cholera depended on the presence of a heat-labile substance as well as the antibodies. This substance, which was first called **alexine**, is now better known as **complement**. By the beginning of the 20th century, it became clear that the same substance was also required for the antibody-mediated lysis of red blood cells. Today, complement has significance for the transfusion scientist for several reasons because it is a substance which is much involved in the pathology of the immune and drug-induced haemolytic anaemias (see Chapter 8), and in blood transfusion reactions (see Chapter 11). In addition, complement is also useful both as a biological reagent in demonstrating the presence of potentially lytic antibodies and to detect clinically significant complement-binding blood group antibodies. This chapter will discuss the activation of complement, its role in immune elimination and its involvement in haemolytic disorders.

3.2 COMPLEMENT IS NOT A SINGLE ENTITY

The name **complement** refers to a set of around 20 different proteins found in the blood plasma and lymph which are able to lyse bacteria and other target cells, including red blood cells. In addition, complement stimulates the inflammatory response, attracts and stimulates neutrophils to engulf these complement-coated cells, and helps to clear the blood and lymph of immune complexes composed of antibody bound to antigen. Thus, complement is important in killing target cells, such as bacteria, and for aiding the immune system in the disposal of the remains by the phagocytic cells. It also stimulates the lysis and phagocytic destruction of antibody-coated red cells in transfusion reactions, haemolytic disease of the newborn and in autoimmune haemolytic anaemias.

Owing to the lytic and inflammatory potential of complement proteins, these proteins are usually present in an inactive form, often as pro-enzymes, requiring conversion into an active enzyme. In other words, complement has to be **activated** to fulfil its role. In addition to the proteins which are involved in these activities, there are a number of proteins which regulate the actions of complement. For example, there are proteins which help to prevent the lysis of the body's own cells, while others prevent excessive activation.

There are three different pathways for the activation of complement. These are known as the **classical**, the **lectin** and the **alternative pathways**. Each of these three activation pathways feeds into a common pathway which results

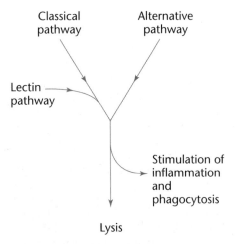

Figure 3.1
Complement may be activated by three different pathways, which converge, causing lysis of a foreign cell and the release of inflammatory mediators. (Courtesy of Micky Hoult, MMU.)

Table 3.1 Activators of complement*

Classical pathway	Alternative pathway
IgG bound to antigen	Lipopolysaccharide (bacterial cell walls)
IgM	Zymosan (yeast cell walls)
C-reactive protein	Heat-aggregated IgA
Heat-aggregated IgG	Trypanosomes
	Cobra venom factor (CVF)
	Some virus-infected cells
	Inulin**

*The lectin pathway is activated by sugar residues on the surface of bacteria.

**Inulin is a polysaccharide obtained from the Jerusalem artichoke! This has very little significance to us *in vivo* but the carbohydrate is often used as an alternative pathway activator *in vitro*.

in the lysis of the target cell. They also each result in the production of proteins which induce phagocytosis and inflammation (see *Fig. 3.1*). The alternative pathway is a first line of defence against microorganisms, because it is activated by the cell wall components of these cells, in the absence of antibody (see *Table 3.1*). This pathway is dependent on the presence of magnesium ions. The classical pathway is initiated when antibody binds to an antigen and may therefore take several days to be effective, if specific antibody is not already present. The classical pathway is dependent on the presence of both magnesium and calcium ions. The lectin pathway does not require the presence of antibody, being stimulated by sugar residues on bacterial cell walls; it feeds into the classical pathway, bypassing the need for antibody.

Box 3.1 Complement terminology

The sequences which involve activation of pro-enzymes are very important to the activity of complement. In such cases, several molecules of a pro-enzyme are cleaved by a previous component in the sequence to yield two fragments, 'a' and 'b', one of which (usually 'b') becomes a new enzyme. There are now several molecules of 'b', each of which is able to cleave many molecules of the next pro-enzyme to yield even more molecules of the next enzyme. Thus, there is amplification in the system. When a complement protein is cleaved into two fragments, 'a' and 'b', on most occasions the 'b' fragment is the largest. The exception to this rule is C2, which is cleaved into a larger C2a and a smaller C2b.

When complement proteins are activated, this is often indicated by a line above the protein, while an inactive form of a previously active component is indicated by the suffix 'i' as in C3bi.

The names 'classical' and 'alternative' may give the impression that the latter is less important than the former. This is not the case because, in terms of speed, the alternative pathway is activated more rapidly, because it does not rely on the presence of antibody. The classical pathway was, in fact, the first to be discovered. The alternative pathway was recognized much later although it is probably more primitive in evolutionary terms. In 1954, Louis Pillemer added zymosan from yeast cell walls to fresh serum and showed that this serum could no longer lyse antibody-coated target cells. This implied that the complement had been 'used up' or **fixed** by something other than antibody.

Table 3.2 Complement proteins

Protein	Molecular mass (kDa)	Pathway
C1q	410	Classical
C1r	190	Classical
C1s	87	Classical
C2	115	Classical and lectin
C3	180	Classical, lectin and alternative
C4	210	Classical and lectin
C5	190	Lytic
C6	128	Lytic
C7	121	Lytic
C8	163	Lytic
C9	79	Lytic
Factor B	93	Alternative
Factor D	24	Alternative
Factor H	150	Alternative
Factor I	88	Alternative
Factor P	220	Alternative
Mannose-binding lectin (MBL)	Oligomer*	Lectin
MASP 1,2,3		Lectin

*MBL subunits are triplets of a 25 kDa glycoprotein. These triplets form oligomers of varying sizes.

The proteins involved in the three activation pathways and in the lytic sequence are shown in *Table 3.2*. Unfortunately, the numbering system does not always follow the chronological sequence of complement activation. It was also discovered, some time after naming, that C1, the first component of complement, was actually a complex of three different proteins and these were subsequently named **C1q**, **C1r** and **C1s**. These proteins are present in the molecular ratio of 1:2:2. They are loosely associated with each other and held together through calcium ions. Complement proteins are produced by a number of cells. The hepatocytes in the liver produce most of the C3, C6, C7, C9 and mannose-binding lectin found in the plasma. During an acute phase response (see Chapter 1), their production is greatly increased. Macrophages produce C1q, C1r and C1s, C2, C4 and C5.

3.3 THE CLASSICAL PATHWAY: ACTIVATION TO LYSIS

The first step in the classical pathway occurs when an antibody binds to an antigen. The only antibodies which can activate complement by this pathway are IgM and IgG. In order to examine complement activation from the point of view of a transfusion scientist, the sequence will be discussed as if an antibody was binding to an antigen on the surface of a red cell. However, this could equally well be happening at the membrane of a bacterial cell. Complement is also activated when antibody binds to a soluble immunogen, such as a toxin, but obviously this will not result in lysis. Instead, the activation of complement leads to clearance of an immune complex, ultimately by the phagocytes.

The complement proteins involved in classical activation are **C1**, **C2**, **C4** and **C3** (in that order) and in the lytic cycle **C5**, **C6**, **C7**, **C8** and **C9**. The starting point for activation of the classical pathway occurs when IgG or IgM binds to an antigen on the red cell membrane. Activation of this pathway requires sufficient antibody to be present on the membrane such that two Fc regions are sufficiently close to bind the same molecule of C1q (see *Fig. 3.2*). IgM is very efficient at activating or **fixing** complement

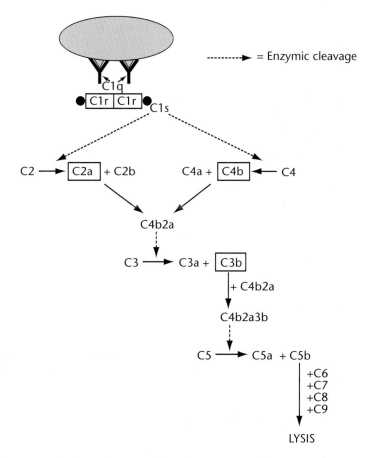

Figure 3.2
Classical pathway for complement activation. Binding of C1q to two adjacent Fc regions on the surface of a red cell initiates a series of reactions, resulting in lysis of the red cells. These reactions are described in the text.

Table 3.3 Blood group antibodies known to bind complement to the red cell membrane

IgM antibodies	IgG antibodies
Anti-A, anti-A$_1$, anti-B	Anti-K
Anti-Le^a, anti-Le^b	Anti-Fy^a
Anti-A$_1$	Anti-Jk^a , anti-Jk^b
Anti-P$_1$	
Anti-H	

because each molecule has five Fc regions close together. IgG, on the other hand, has only one Fc region per molecule and it has been estimated that approximately 1000 molecules of IgG must bind to a red cell in order to achieve the density required for activation to occur. A list of IgM and IgG antibodies relevant to transfusion is shown in *Table 3.3*.

Box 3.2 IgG subclasses and complement activation

In Chapter 2, it was explained that IgG exists in four subclasses each with different properties. These differences extend to their ability to activate complement. Thus, IgG$_3$ activates complement more effectively than IgG$_1$, while IgG$_2$ is much less effective and IgG$_4$ does not activate complement at all. Thus, a blood group antibody which is of the IgG$_4$ subclass will not be detected by methods which depend on complement binding.

C1q is a large protein (see *Table 3.2* and *Fig. 3.3*). Its three-dimensional structure, seen on electron micrographs, has been likened to a bunch of six tulips which are all fused at the stalks. Each of the 'flowers' is able to bind to a site on the Fc region of the antibody. The site to which the C1q binds is located on the C_H2 domain of IgG and the C_H3 domain of IgM (see Chapter 2). All that is required to activate complement is for two of the 'tulip heads' to become bound to adjacent Fc regions at the red cell membrane. This binding is facilitated by the 'tulip stalks', which contain collagen-like protein sequences and are very flexible.

The binding of C1q in this manner results in the activation of the C1r component. C1r acquires enzymatic activity and cleaves a peptide from C1s to expose the active site of this proteolytic enzyme.

Activated C1s is a proteolytic enzyme. It is able to cleave C4 into two fragments, C4a and C4b. C4b has a hydrophobic binding site which allows it to bind to the red cell membrane. It binds at membrane sites other than those already occupied by antibody. This is only a transient binding site. Any C4b which fails to bind to the red cell continues the sequence in the plasma.

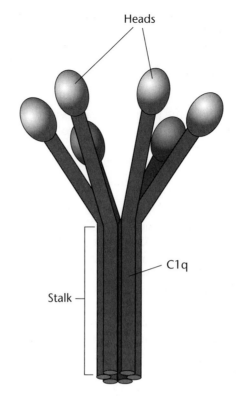

Figure 3.3
The C1q molecule (courtesy of Micky Hoult, MMU).

C1s also acts on the next complement component, C2, and cleaves it into two fragments: C2a and C2b. The larger fragment, C2a, binds to C4b at the red cell membrane in the presence of magnesium ions to form a new enzyme, **C4b2a**. The smaller fragments, C4a and C2b, remain in the plasma. The new enzyme C4b2a is otherwise known as the **classical pathway C3 convertase** because it is capable of cleaving C3 into two fragments, C3a and C3b.

Box 3.3 The lytic action of complement requires activated complement proteins to attach to the cell surface

Prior to activation all complement proteins are dissolved in the plasma, i.e. the fluid phase.

In order to lyse a cell, complement proteins have to be recruited onto the membrane of the target cell. There are several steps in the activation process in which complement proteins are taken out of the fluid phase and recruited to the target cell membrane, the first being when C1q binds to the Fc region of the antibody, which is itself bound to the target cell membrane. At other stages, activated complement proteins acquire transient hydrophobic binding sites that allow them to attach to the membrane phospholipids.

C3b contains most of the structure of C3, with the exception of a 9000 Da fragment (C3a) cleaved from one of the two polypeptide chains which make up this protein. C3a has significant inflammatory properties, which are discussed below. When first produced, C3b, like C4b, has a transient binding site that allows it to bind to the red cell membrane or to the C3 convertase C4b2a. C3b which fails to bind to the membrane continues the sequence in the plasma. The presence of a very short-term binding site helps to ensure that C3b only binds to cells close to its production. This is most likely to be the 'target' cell to which the C1q has become bound. Binding of C3b to 'self' cells would ultimately result in injury to those cells.

Whether it is attached to the red cell or not, a molecule of C3b which binds to a molecule of the C3 convertase (C4b2a) produces a new enzyme, **C4b2aC3b**, which is a **C5 convertase**. This enzyme cleaves C5 into two fragments: C5a and C5b. C5a has inflammatory properties which will be discussed later. C5b also has a transient hydrophobic binding site which allows it to bind to the target cell membrane. At this stage, the red cell has numerous proteins attached to the membrane at different sites. These proteins include antibody, C1q, C4b, C4b2a, C3b, C4b2aC3b and C5b (see *Fig. 3.4*). All steps up to this stage are enzymic and much amplification occurs, so that there may be thousands of molecules of C5b attached to the membrane. The pores in the membrane which will eventually result in haemolysis are produced at the sites where C5b has bound.

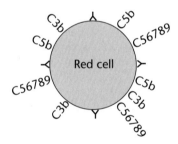

Figure 3.4
Consequences of complement activation. A red cell coated with antibody becomes coated with a variety of complement proteins, each with biological activity. Moreover, there are far more of these molecules on the red cell than molecules of the antibody which triggered activation, i.e. amplification has occurred.

Box 3.4 The presence of complement on red cells infers the presence of antibody

When an antibody-coated red blood cell becomes coated with complement proteins following complement activation, there is very much more complement on the red blood cell than the antibody which triggered it in the first place. This is due to amplification which occurs when complement proteins become enzymic following activation. Therefore, in a transfusion laboratory, it is always much easier to detect complement on red blood cells than to detect antibodies. The presence of activated complement proteins on red blood cells is used as an indicator of the presence of complement-binding antibodies.

The following stages are not enzymic, but instead involve the addition, sequentially, to C5b, of a molecule each of C6, C7 and C8 and several copies of C9. This produces a large molecule, known as the **membrane attack complex (MAC)** with a RMM of more than 10^6 Da. Each MAC is built up at the membrane as a set of hydrophobic proteins lining a cylinder. The cylinder becomes inserted into the membrane of the target cells and a pore is produced. The pores themselves have a diameter of approximately 10 nm. They allow the passage of ions and small molecules to occur between the cell and its environment such that the normal gradients of these molecules across the cell membrane are lost, and equilibration occurs. However, because large molecules such as proteins are too big to leak out of the cell, a high osmotic pressure is built up within the cell, allowing water to cross the undamaged membrane by osmosis. This influx of water kills the cell.

Lysis of antibody-coated cells is most spectacularly seen with red cells, which literally burst following the activation of the classical pathway. *In vitro*, this can be seen a sudden 'clearing' of a previously cloudy cell suspension, due to the release of haemoglobin from the cells. With other types of mammalian cell, the reaction is not so dramatic and the cells die without necessarily bursting immediately. These cells can be shown to be dead by staining them with dyes which are normally excluded from cells with intact, healthy membranes (see tissue typing in Chapter 12).

Box 3.5 Reactive lysis

Any C5b which fails to bind to the membrane can continue the sequence in the fluid phase. There is the possibility that complexes of C5b67 can bind to innocent bystander cells and initiate lysis. Such a situation is called reactive lysis. Reactive lysis may amplify the effects of any unwanted antibody, such as an antibody to red blood cells. *In vivo*, red cells are resistant to reactive lysis owing to the presence of membrane inhibitors, such as CD59.

3.4 OTHER BIOLOGICAL ACTIVITIES OF COMPLEMENT

The lytic activity of complement is not its major defence role *in vivo*, even though it is a very useful end point in *in vitro* assays and, as previously mentioned, plays a strong part in the pathology of transfusion reactions and haemolytic anaemias. Other important roles of complement include stimulation of phagocytosis through the attraction of phagocytes and promotion of opsonization, stimulation of inflammation and the clearance of immune complexes. These non-lytic activities of complement may be more significant in the beneficial role of complement in eliminating microorganisms from the body. They may also have significant effects during transfusion reactions.

Activated complement may also react with other systems, including the blood clotting and fibrinolytic systems. Interaction with the former promotes the aggregation of platelets and may contribute to the pathology of transfusion reactions. Interaction with the fibrinolytic system promotes the dissolution of blood clots. The reader who wishes to learn more about the wealth of complement activities is advised to see the recommended reading at the end of this chapter.

Attraction of phagocytes, opsonization and clearance of immune complexes

The proteins C3a and C5a are chemotactic for neutrophils. This means that neutrophils will be attracted to any area where complement is activated. It is this activity that is thought to play a significant role in the build up of neutrophils at a site of inflammation, particularly when bacteria have entered that site. The complex C5b67 is also known to be chemotactic for neutrophils.

Phagocytic cells, including neutrophils, monocytes and macrophages, have receptors for C3b. Thus, a cell which has become coated with C3b will bind to these receptors, a phenomenon known as **immune adherence**. C3b-coated red cells may also bind to surfaces such as the walls of blood vessels, making them easy targets for phagocytic cells in the blood. There are various forms of complement receptor (CR) which bind C3b and its derivatives (see *Table 3.4*).

Table 3.4 Complement receptors

Receptor	Complement proteins bound	Distribution
CR1	C3b, C4b, C3bi*	Red cells, eosinophils, neutrophils, monocytes, macrophages, B cells, some T cells, follicular dendritic cells (in lymph nodes)
CR2	C3bi, C3dg*, C3d*	B cells, follicular dendritic cells
CR3	C3bi	Neutrophils, NK cells, monocytes, macrophages, follicular dendritic cells
CR4	C3bi	Neutrophils, monocytes, macrophages, platelets

*These proteins are various forms of inactivated C3b. They are discussed with the **alternative pathway**.

Binding of the complement-coated cell to the phagocyte in this way activates the phagocyte so that it is more efficient at ingesting and destroying cell. The metabolism of the phagocyte is also enhanced. C3b can also become bound to soluble immune complexes, favouring their binding to, and subsequent uptake by, the phagocytes. Red blood cells also have CR1 receptors in their membranes so that C3b-coated cells bind to circulating red blood cells and are removed by phagocytes in the liver and the spleen. Each red blood cell has far fewer CR1 receptor molecules per cell than a phagocyte, but this does not mean that their role is insignificant, because there are approximately 1000 red blood cells for every leucocyte. It has been calculated that, collectively, red blood cells have 90% of the CR1 molecules in the blood and are therefore very important in removing immune complexes from the blood stream.

Stimulation of inflammation

C3a, C5a and, to a lesser extent, C4a have **anaphylatoxin** activity. This means that they bind to blood basophils and tissue mast cells and cause them to degranulate. The chemicals released include histamine, which causes vasodilation, thus allowing more plasma, containing complement and antibodies, to get into the inflamed site. In addition, the dilated blood vessel allows the neutrophils to gain access to the site to which they have been chemotactically attracted. It is also known that C5a binds to macrophages, inducing them to release interleukin (IL)-1 and IL-6, both of which are known to increase the expression of **cell adhesion molecules (CAM)** on the surface of the endothelial cells which line the blood vessel. These CAM are necessary for the adherence of neutrophils to the blood vessel and for their migration between the endothelial cells and into the inflamed site. In addition, IL-1 and IL-6 stimulate the bone marrow to release neutrophil reserves during an acute phase response. Thus, it can be seen that all the different responses to damage and infection are very much interrelated.

3.5 ALTERNATIVE PATHWAY FOR COMPLEMENT ACTIVATION

The alternative pathway for complement activation is actually not a pathway at all: it is a **positive feedback loop**. This is an amplification system which increases C3 breakdown, whenever C3b has been produced. An alternative pathway activator can then be seen as anything which increases the activity of this 'loop'. This amplification loop, and its regulation, is shown in *Fig. 3.5*.

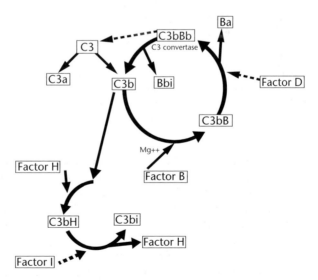

Figure 3.5
The alternative pathway for complement activation. The alternative pathway involves a positive amplification loop in which C3b positively stimulates the breakdown of more C3. Details of this pathway and its control are described in the text.

Whenever C3b has been produced, perhaps from the classical pathway, or perhaps by a very slow natural breakdown of C3 into C3a and C3b, this C3b can enter the amplification loop. The protein Factor B, which is present in plasma, binds to C3b to form a complex, C3bB. The Factor B which forms part of this complex is then cleaved by a plasma enzyme known as Factor D, releasing the smaller fragment, Ba, and leaving Bb as part of the complex: C3bBb. This complex is the **alternative pathway C3 convertase** and catalyses the cleavage of more C3 into C3a and C3b. If this feedback loop were uncontrolled, then the plasma content of C3 would very rapidly be exhausted due to its breakdown and more and more C3b would appear on cell surfaces. However, there are several control points. For example, C3bBb is an inherently unstable enzyme and breaks down to produce C3b and an inactive form of Bb (Bbi). In addition, there is a regulatory loop in which C3b becomes bound to Factor H, another plasma protein. C3bH is then susceptible to an enzyme, Factor I, which converts C3b to an inactive form (C3bi) which can no longer enter the amplification loop.

Alternative pathway activators are generally macromolecules which stabilize the C3bBb enzyme. They may do this by forming a protective surface to which the enzyme adheres, and where it is less susceptible to breaking down. Macromolecules which act as alternative pathway activators are often very long molecules with a highly repetitive structure, seemingly making a highly stabilizing surface.

Bacteria are also known to activate Factor P (properdin), a plasma globulin, such that it changes configuration to one which provides a stabilizing surface.

Cobra venom factor (CVF) is a very well-known alternative pathway activator that works in a somewhat different way. CVF is a molecule with a structure rather similar to C3b. Thus, CVF enters the amplification loop, eventually being responsible for extensive C3 cleavage. However, CVF does not bind to Factor H and cannot be inactivated by Factor I and is therefore not regulated by this loop. The injection of CVF into an animal causes a rapid loss of C3 in plasma as it eventually all gets cleaved by the convertase enzyme.

The alternative pathway can feed into the lytic sequence

C3b, the product of the alternative pathway, can also feed into the common lytic sequence, resulting in lysis of microorganisms. This happens when a molecule of C3b binds to the alternative pathway convertase, to form a new enzyme, **C3bBbC3b**, which is a C5 convertase. From this point, the two activation pathways merge.

3.6 THE LECTIN PATHWAY

This pathway is activated when mannose-binding lectin (MBL) binds to sugar residues on the surface of bacteria. The binding to bacteria promotes the binding, and subsequent activation, of MBL-associated proteases (MASP) such as MASP1 and MASP2. These proteins cleave C4 into C4a and C4b, and

C2 into C2a and C2b. The subsequent steps are identical to those of the classical pathway (see above). Thus, MBL provides a means for activating the classical pathway in the absence of antibody. This pathway is particularly important in young children, who may not have acquired specific immunity to a wide range of bacterial infections.

3.7 PHYSIOLOGICAL REGULATION OF COMPLEMENT ACTIVATION

In its physiological role, careful regulation of complement activity is required in order to prevent damage to the body, particularly from lytic and inflammatory mediators. Factors H and I are important regulators of C3b production and disposal. Inactive C3b (C3bi) produced by the action of these two proteins is further degraded into smaller fragments, C3dg and C3d, which remain bound to the coated red blood cell. In addition, any C4b which has bound to a red blood cell is degraded to a smaller fragment, C4d, which remains bound. Many potentially lytic anti-red cell antibodies do not proceed to lysis *in vitro* owing to the presence of natural regulators. Therefore, instead of looking for lysis as an end point of complement activation, the transfusion scientist will look for the presence of cell-bound C3d, using an appropriate antibody.

Some molecules known to regulate complement are shown in *Table 3.5*. Deficiency of any of these regulators may result in chronic activation of complement.

3.8 COMPLEMENT IN TRANSFUSION SCIENCE

A serum containing anti-red blood cell antibodies, particularly of the IgM class, has the potential to cause haemolysis by activation of complement.

Table 3.5 Regulators of complement activity

Regulator/name	Role
C1INH/C1 inhibitor	Inhibits the action of C1r on C1s and C1s on its substrate
C3bINA/C3b inactivator	Splits cell-bound and fluid-phase C3b into two fragments, C3c and C3dg, the latter then being degraded further to yield C3d. This effectively destroys the C5 convertase of both pathways and the independent biological activities of C3b
Carboxypeptidase B	Inhibits the anaphylatoxin activities of C3a and C5a
DAF/Decay accelerating factor	Interacts with C4b and C3b so as to allow Factor I to cleave them
Factors H and I	Remove C3b from the amplification loop and convert it to the inactive C3bi

This is true in transfusion reactions (e.g. anti-A, anti-B) as well as in sera with auto-antibodies against red blood cells. Detection of these antibodies is essential. Such antibodies may be detected by haemolysis, using complement, or they may be detected by looking for activated complement proteins coating the surface of red blood cells with which the serum has been incubated.

Establishing complement levels of sera

Occasionally it might be necessary to establish that a serum has normal complement activity. This might be needed, for example, when wishing to detect antibodies to red cells by complement-dependent lysis rather than the more usual agglutination. In such cases, sheep red blood cells coated with a sub-agglutinating level of anti-sheep red blood cell antibodies are used. Such cells are commonly known as **sensitized sheep red cells**. Serial dilutions of the serum are incubated with sensitized cells and the amount of haemolysis compared with a set of standards to assess the percentage haemolysis, and thus the amount of complement. A serum which has a complement level of less than 50% of normal is likely to be unsatisfactory for the detection of complement-fixing antibodies.

Loss of complement activity in sera

Loss of complement can sometimes affect the activity of a serum in demonstrating haemolysis. Factors which diminish complement activity in sera with previously normal complement levels include heat, incorrect storage and the presence of some anticoagulants. In addition, some sera show anti-complement activity.

Inactivation by heating. Complement is heat-labile and all complement activity is lost when serum is heated to 56°C for 30 minutes. Heating serum in this way is a standard method for effectively removing complement from a sample. This might be necessary, for example, when trying to demonstrate agglutination, or when standardizing complement levels in sera by first heating and then adding a standard amount of complement from a known source. It should be noted that heating serum at 37°C for 1 hour will also inactivate complement so care should be taken when thawing frozen sera at this temperature, if complement activity is to be retained.

Incorrect storage. Sera should be stored at −20°C to retain complement activity. However, sera which have been exposed to repeated cycles of freezing and thawing, or have been kept at room temperature for long periods, will soon lose their complement activity.

Anticoagulants. Both heparin and EDTA can inhibit complement. EDTA is the worst offender since it is a chelating agent and calcium and magnesium are both required for classical activation. This may present problems when wishing to use plasma, rather than serum, to detect potentially lytic antibodies.

Anti-complementary activity. Some sera may have anti-complementary activity which inhibits the action of complement. Examples of this include sera with raised or abnormal immunoglobulin levels, and sera which have been incorrectly stored and contain a denatured and inactive form of complement known as **complementoid**.

Complement-deficient sera may be restored by the addition of fresh ABO-compatible serum which has been pooled from a number of samples. Test sera containing anti-complementary activity may be first incubated with red blood cells to allow binding of potentially lytic antibodies; the cells are then washed and pooled fresh serum is added as a source of complement.

Significance of complement binding by anti-red blood cell antibodies

Antibodies to red blood cells may be drug-induced, autoimmune, or antibodies to blood group antigens (see Chapters 5 and 6). All IgM antibodies bind complement efficiently and are therefore potentially highly lytic *in vivo* and *in vitro* (although, as previously mentioned, red blood cells do not usually bind sufficient complement to cause haemolysis *in vitro*). Examples of red blood cell antibodies which are of the IgM class include anti-A and anti-B and antibodies to the Lewis blood group. In autoimmune haemolytic disorders, antibodies are frequently IgG. Other blood groups in which IgG anti-red cell antibodies predominate include Duffy and Kell. In these cases, complement activation may or may not result, depending on the IgG subclass, the number of antigenic sites and the affinity of the antibody.

Non-lytic complement-fixing antibodies

Tests for haemolytic antibodies in sera invariably rely on the presence of sufficient antibody to give optimum conditions for lysis of red blood cells following the antigen/antibody reaction. If there is insufficient antibody, as is often the case, the antigen/antibody complex may fix sub-haemolytic doses of complement. In such cases, the red blood cells become coated with the most stable components of the complement reaction, i.e. the C3dg and C4d components. These may be detected by using antibodies to these components to stimulate not lysis but haemagglutination. This technique is discussed in further detail in Chapter 10.

Complement deficiencies

Inherited deficiencies of nearly all the complement components have been found in humans. Deficiencies in C3, MBL, Factor H and Factor I lead to increased susceptibility to infection, especially with pyogenic (pus-producing) bacteria. Deficiencies in C1, C4 and C2 are associated with the development of immune complex disorders such as **systemic lupus erythematosus**, an autoimmune disease in which immune complexes persist in organs such as the kidney and cause inflammatory reactions wherever they are deposited, and vasculitis. Deficiencies in the proteins involved in the lytic sequence and Factors D and P lead to increases in susceptibility to *Neisseria meningitidis* and *N. gonorrhoea*. Deficiency of the regulatory protein C1INH (see *Table 3.5*) results in **hereditary angioneurotic oedema**, a condition characterized by episodes of inflammatory swelling in different parts of the body.

Deficiencies of the complement proteins involved in lysis, such as C5, C6, C7 and C8, lead to recurrent and severe neisserial infections, particularly *N. meningitidis*, which causes meningitis.

Box 3.6 Paroxysmal nocturnal haemoglobinuria – a rare disease

Paroxysmal nocturnal haemoglobinuria (PNH) is a rare syndrome, usually diagnosed in patients when they are investigated for the presence of free haemoglobin in the urine. One of the first symptoms is that of dark brown urine on waking, which gradually returns to normal as the day continues. Sometimes it continues for a few days at a time, hence its name. However, the syndrome was also noticed in shift workers who were awake at night but sleeping in the daytime, thus suggesting that the 'nocturnal' aspect was a misnomer. Testing of the blood revealed that the red cells, which are haemolysing and being excreted in the urine, were in fact overly sensitive to complement. During sleep, the body's pH levels are reduced and this acid environment causes complement to bind to red cells and haemolysis results. The resulting symptoms include anaemia, thrombosis and sometimes bone marrow failure leading to 'aplastic anaemia', in which very few blood cells are produced. PNH is due to an X-linked genetic mutation which prevents proteins attaching to the red cell membrane. The gene affected is the phosphatidylinositol glycan A (*PIG A*) gene encoding a protein required to make the glycosyl phosphatidylinositol (GPI) molecule, which acts as an anchor for many red cell membrane proteins. The complement-related proteins CD55 (also known as decay accelerating factor, or DAF) and CD59 (membrane inhibitor of reacting lysis, or MIRL) both require this GPI anchor for their expression on the red cell membrane. The lack of the GPI anchor means that these inhibitors of complement-mediated lysis are lacking and so the patient's red cells are more susceptible to complement-mediated lysis. Other blood cells are also affected; the involvement of platelets causes them to clump in the blood vessels resulting in thrombosis.

SUGGESTED FURTHER READING

Engelfreit, C.P. (1992) The immune destruction of red cells. *Transfusion Medicine* **2**, 1–6.

Lambris, J.D. (ed.) (2006) Current topics in complement. *Advances in Experimental Medicine and Biology* **586**, 1–393.

Lambris, J.D. and Holers, V.M. (eds) (2000) *Therapeutic Interventions in the Complement System*. New Jersey: Humana.

Rother, K., Till, G.O. and Hansch, G.M. (eds) (1998) *The Complement System*, 2nd edn. Berlin: Springer.

Turner, M.W. (2003) The role of mannose-binding lectin in health and disease. *Molecular Immunology* **40**, 423–429.

Volanakis, J.E. and Frank, M.M. (eds) (1998) *The Human Complement System in Health and Disease*. New York: Marcel Decker.

Walport, M.J. (2001) Complement. First of two parts. *New England Journal of Medicine* **344**, 1058–1066.

Walport, M.J. (2001) Complement. Second of two parts. *New England Journal of Medicine* **344**, 1140–1144.

SELF-ASSESSMENT QUESTIONS

1. Which class of antibodies is most efficient at activating complement?
2. Why is there more complement on a red cell than the antibody which activated complement?
3. How do complement proteins in plasma end up on the membrane of an antibody-coated red cell?
4. Describe what is meant by an anaphylatoxin. In what way do they stimulate phagocytosis?
5. How may complement levels in serum be assessed in the laboratory?
6. Describe a laboratory method for inactivating complement.
7. Why is EDTA a problem when demonstrating antibody-induced haemolysis?

Genetics for blood groups

Learning objectives
After studying this chapter you should be able to:

■ Define some of the significant terms relating to genetics

■ Describe the nature of DNA and chromosomes

■ Define the gene as a unit of genetic material

■ Understand how the Mendelian laws of genetics relate to blood group inheritance

■ Describe the difference between the terms 'genotype' and 'phenotype'

■ Distinguish between types of inheritance, including autosomal, co-dominant, sex-linked, dominant and recessive

■ Discuss the significance and contribution of molecular genetics to blood groups

4.1 GENETICS AND BLOOD GROUPS

It is essential to understand genetics in relation to blood groups in order to appreciate the issues involved in typing the blood group of an individual or selecting blood for transfusion purposes. Blood group systems are inherited and are known to have either a single gene (the majority), or two or more genes, which are closely linked on a chromosome. A discussion of the terms involved in genetics (from the Greek word meaning 'to generate') follows. Most of the initial discoveries about how hereditary information is passed down generations were first made by Mendel and published in 1865. The many discoveries in the first half of the 20th century concerning the nature of the genetic material culminated in the work of Watson and Crick in 1953. They gave a clear insight into the structure of the genetic material, deoxyribonucleic acid (DNA), and how inheritance might occur. The explosion of information in the area of molecular biology, which has been central to the development of biology in modern times, has been extensively used in transfusion science. Indeed, modern techniques have been applied to expand knowledge of the inheritance and nature of blood group antigens and a wealth of literature is available in this area. Currently, the genes encoding almost all of the 23 blood group systems have been cloned and sequenced. This chapter includes a brief overview of traditional genetics, combined with more recent findings relating to blood group systems.

4.2   DNA AND CHROMOSOMES

The human body is composed of somatic (body) cells, the nuclei of which each contain 23 pairs of chromosomes: 22 pairs of **autosomes** and one set of sex chromosomes, either XX (if female) or XY (if male). The pairs are **homologous**, meaning that they contain the same genes at the same locations. Cells which have the complete set of 23 pairs of chromosomes are called **diploid**. During sexual reproduction, gametes (ova and spermatozoa) are produced which each have half the number of chromosomes, i.e. they are **haploid**. These cells have one chromosome from each homologous pair and one sex chromosome. As a result of fertilization, a diploid cell is produced, which gives rise to the embryo. Thus, any individual inherits half their chromosomes from their mother and half from their father (see Section 4.6 for more details about inheritance).

Each chromosome consists of a single long molecule of DNA. Each DNA molecule is made up of two very long polynucleotide strands running in opposite directions (i.e. they are **anti-parallel**). The nucleotides that make up each strand consist of an organic, nitrogenous base, which is either a purine or a pyrimidine, a deoxyribose sugar and a phosphate group. The nucleotides are joined together by links between the phosphate of one nucleotide and the sugar of the next (the phosphodiester bond). Thus, the backbone of each strand is sugar–phosphate–sugar–phosphate, etc. while the nitrogenous base forms the step of a 'ladder' at right angles to the backbone. The second strand is 'upside down' with respect to the first, bringing the two organic bases close together so that hydrogen bonds can form between them. There are four bases found in DNA: the purines **adenine** (**A**) and **guanine** (**G**), and the pyrimidines **thymine** (**T**) and **cytosine** (**C**). They 'pair up' in a precise manner with adenine binding, through hydrogen bonds, to thymine and guanine to cytosine. The double-stranded DNA is then twisted into the characteristic double helix. The sequence of nucleotides in the DNA strand is extremely important because it is a code containing the information required for the synthesis of RNA and protein. Blood group, or red cell, antigens consist of either membrane proteins, or of carbohydrate structures conferred on the red cells by the activity of enzymes, which again are proteins. Thus, an understanding of protein synthesis is important (see Section 4.4). It is crucial to understand that the wide diversity of antigens found in human blood groups is ultimately determined at the level of information carried by the genes.

4.3   THE STRUCTURE AND ROLE OF GENES

A gene was defined in 1909 by Johannsen as a hereditary factor that constitutes a single unit of hereditary material, which is part of a chromosome.

Genes code for proteins, which in blood group terms means either a polypeptide chain consisting of a specific amino acid sequence, or an enzyme, for example a transferase, which transfers a monosaccharide (sugar) onto a substrate consisting of other molecules or structures in the red blood cell membrane. Structurally, genes are segments of the linear DNA strand which makes up the chromosome. The genes are a sequence of nucleotides which encode the amino acid sequence of a protein. A sequence of three nucleotides encodes a single amino acid. This triplet sequence is called a **codon**. There are 64 different ways in which nucleotides containing the four bases can be combined to form triplets. Thus, there are more than enough coding sequences to encode the 20 or so different amino acids which are found in proteins. In fact, a single amino acid may be encoded by more than one triplet, for example ACA and ACC both code for threonine. Other triplets are regulatory codons, for example, for stopping the transcription of DNA. These are known as stop codons. The sequences of nucleotides which encode amino acids are called **exons**, while the sequences that do not are called **introns**. Although the DNA encodes a sequence of amino acids, DNA is first transcribed into messenger RNA (mRNA) in the nucleus, and is then 'translated' into protein on the ribosomes in the cytoplasm. This 'arrangement' both ensures that the DNA remains within the nucleus, and also allows for additional control over protein synthesis, which can be controlled at the transcription and translation stages.

The position of the genes on the chromosome is called the **locus** (plural **loci**). When genes exist in alternative forms at the same locus on homologous chromosomes, they are known as **alleles**. The proteins produced by allelic genes may be structurally similar, but even small differences create different antigenic sites. Some blood group antigens are amino acid sequences which give rise to a specific blood group. It is interesting to note that the substitution of just one amino acid can result in a difference in

Table 4.1 Some examples of amino acid substitutions which result in blood group specificity

Blood group	Antigen	Amino acid	Nucleotide
MNS	M → N	Ser → Leu	C → T
		Gly → Glu	G → A
	S → s	Met → Thr	T → C
Lutheran	Lu^a → Lu^b	His → Arg	A → G
Kidd	Jk^a → Jk^b	Asp → Asn	G → A
Duffy	Fy^a → Fy^b	Gly → Asp	G → A
Rh	C → c	Ser → Pro	T → C
		Ile → Leu	A → C
		Ser → Asn	G → A
	E → e	Pro → Ala	C → G

blood group specificity; for some examples see *Table 4.1*. An example of this in a blood group system is the *RHCE* gene of the Rh system, which has multiple alleles encoding antigens C, c, E and e (see Chapter 6). The *KEL* gene, which is responsible for the Kell blood group system, shows a high degree of **polymorphism**. Thus, it possesses a number of alleles, each encoding the expression of different epitopes (see Chapter 2 for a definition of 'epitopes'). For more details of the Kell blood group system, see Chapter 7.

4.4 DNA REPLICATION AND PROTEIN SYNTHESIS

Before a somatic cell divides, replication of the DNA strand must occur in order to provide the same complement of DNA for the new cells formed by mitosis. This process involves the two DNA strands unwinding, a process controlled by the helicase enzyme. Each new strand then acts as a template for the formation of a new complementary chain. During protein synthesis, DNA partially unwinds and portions act as a template for the synthesis of a single-stranded ribonucleic acid (RNA). This messenger RNA (mRNA) is complementary to the DNA region copied and, like all RNA molecules, contains ribose instead of deoxyribose and the pyrimidine uracil instead of thymine.

This process of mRNA production, using DNA as a template, is known as **transcription**. The enzyme DNA polymerase is involved in the process by attaching to the DNA molecule and opening a strand of the double helix. Thus, transcription of DNA occurs as the nascent mRNA peels away from the DNA strand. This RNA is then transferred from the nucleus to the cytoplasm and attaches to ribosomes, which are the site of protein synthesis. At the ribosomes, the amino acids, which are free in the cell pool, are brought to the ribosomes by transfer RNA (tRNA). Each amino acid is attached to a specific tRNA containing a sequence of bases which is complementary to the codon and is called the **anti-codon**. This tRNA then attaches to mRNA and brings along with it the appropriate amino acid. As the amino acids are joined together by peptide bonds, a polypeptide chain is produced. This may be further modified within the cell by the addition of carbohydrates and lipids (post-translational modification). The process of protein synthesis is depicted in *Fig. 4.1*.

4.5 BLOOD GROUPS AND MOLECULAR EVENTS IN GENES

A variety of molecular mechanisms causes the diversity of blood group antigens to be formed, including point mutation, deletion or insertion of nucleotides, altered splicing events, gene crossover and gene conversion. As the sequence of bases in DNA contains the code for a protein, any change in that sequence will alter the nature of the protein produced. Sometimes mutations, or substitutions of single bases within the codon, occur spontaneously. The effect of a mutation is to change the codon and hence the amino acid in the protein. There are several different types of mutation, which have varying effects on the protein produced.

a) Transcription

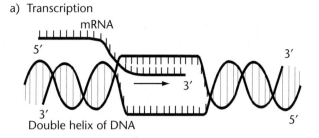

b) Translation

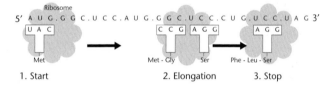

c) Stages of translation

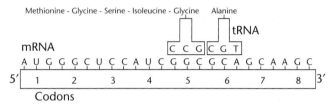

Figure 4.1
Stages in protein synthesis.

Silent mutations may occur because there are several codons for the same amino acid. Thus, a change from ACA, which codes for threonine, to ACC will still result in the code for threonine. Sometimes an amino acid is substituted for another but this has no evident effect on the phenotype; again this is a silent mutation.

Missense mutations involve substitutions of bases, resulting in a change in the amino acid sequence and giving rise to an abnormal protein product.

Frameshift mutations occur when there is a deletion or insertion of one or more bases into the codon sequence. As the code is read in triplets, this results in the reading frame being altered. A good example of this is blood group O. Studies have shown that the DNA sequence of the O allele is the same as that for the A allele except that a single base is deleted at the 258 position. The resulting transferase enzyme is non-functional (see Chapter 5).

Other blood group antigens have resulted from DNA mutations. For example, the MNS blood group system includes the S antigen, which contains the amino acid methionine, encoded by the nucleotide sequence ATG. If the code is altered to ACG, threonine is incorporated instead of methionine, giving rise to the s antigen. Gene duplication is shown in the Rh system, which has the genes *RHD* and *RHCE* together on chromosome 1. The Rh blood group is interesting in that the two genes are very similar, i.e. they are highly homologous and each gene has ten exons. The genes each encode a polypeptide chain which is 417 amino acids in length, but differing slightly in amino acid constitution. Other genetic events which occur in blood groups are single crossover, gene conversion, transcriptional errors and splicing errors. Splicing errors occur when the specific motifs at the 3′ and 5′ ends of the introns are altered by a nucleotide change. This results in exon skipping, an example of which is seen in the the Jk(a–b–) phenotype of the Kidd blood group.

Molecular biology techniques, which involve a study of the structure, replication and expression of genes, have been crucial in developing an understanding of the genetics of blood groups, in particular how they are produced, and how they are inherited by individuals. Chapter 13 describes molecular aspects in more detail and gives some applications of these techniques.

Box 4.1 Some useful terms

Exons	The coding parts of a gene
Introns	Sequences between the exons
Transcription	Creation of RNA from a gene sequence, yielding mRNA
Point mutation	Change of a single nucleotide in the coding region of DNA
Translation	The use of information from mRNA to make a new protein
Codon	Groups of three nucleotides in a specific order
Stop codon	Signal for the end of translation
Open reading frame	Region between the start and stop codons
Frameshift	Insertion or deletion of nucleotides resulting in alterations in gene length and the subsequent sequence of codons
Insertion	Gain of a single nucleotide or segment of DNA
Deletion	Loss of a single nucleotide or segment of DNA
Single crossover	Exchange of part of a gene from one chromosome with the partner chromosome

---

4.6 INHERITANCE OF BLOOD GROUP GENES

Individuals inherit one set of chromosomes from their mother and one from their father. The testes in men and the ovaries in women are the site of production of cells containing a haploid set of chromosomes. These cells are known as **gametes** and are the ova in women or spermatozoa in men. During fertilization of the ovum by the spermatozoa, the two haploid nuclei fuse together to form diploid cells. Thus, the developing embryo has 23 pairs of chromosomes again. The inheritance of chromosomes and the genes within them is governed by the Mendelian laws of genetics.

Mendelian laws and patterns of inheritance

Mendel's findings have become the basis of inheritance patterns. The laws of segregation, independent assortment and dependent assortment of genetically determined traits are applicable to the inheritance of blood groups.

The law of **segregation** refers to the separation of a single pair of genes on homologous chromosomes when they pass to different gametes during the process of meiosis. The law of **independent assortment** states that genes which are not on homologous chromosomes or are situated far apart on homologous chromosomes separate independently and that the complement of chromosomes passed to the sex cell is governed by chance. The genes are not linked together so they separate independently. **Dependent assortment**, or **linkage**, states that genes on the same chromosome with gene loci which are close together are inherited together and are said to be 'linked'. Linkage is seen in genes of the HLA/major histocompatibility complex (see Chapters 1 and 12). As a result, the genes do not segregate independently and if positioned close together are unlikely to be separated by the process of crossing over which also occurs in meiosis. **Crossing over** is a process by which two homologous chromosomes exchange part of their DNA during meiosis. Thus, nucleotides are interchanged between chromosomes and two recombinants are generated as a result. This allows the recombination of genetic material in future offspring. An example of the effect of crossing over is seen in the genes which code for glycophorin A and glycophorin B, the carbohydrate substances responsible for the MNS blood group system. The MNS blood group system is further described in Chapter 7.

Zygosity: homozygous and heterozygous

When a zygote inherits two identical alleles of a gene at a particular locus, the zygote is said to be **homozygous** for that gene. When the alleles are different, the zygote is **heterozygous** for that gene. In blood grouping terms, a homozygous individual has more antigen sites for a particular blood group than one who is heterozygous. This is referred to as a **dosage effect** and is seen in laboratory tests when red cells give a stronger agglutination reaction when tested with a corresponding antibody. Therefore, homozygous individuals exhibit a 'double dose' of the gene product, which in this instance refers to specific blood group antigens, whilst heterozygotes have only a single dose. An example of a blood group which exhibits dosage effects in laboratory tests is the Rh group (see Chapter 6). The mating of heterozygous individuals may result in a homozygous recessive trait being inherited, for example parents, each of whom are heterozygous for the *A* allele of the *ABO* gene (genotype AO), may produce a child who is homozygous for blood group A and a child who is blood group O. Here is another example: heterozygous parents carrying an inactive *FUT1* (*H*) gene allele, that is, one normal and one inactive gene for the production of H sugar, may produce an offspring who is homozygous for an inactive *FUT1* gene. This is the genetic basis of the rare **Bombay phenotype**, which is described in Chapter 5. Zygosity is also of importance in considering inherited diseases, such as haemophilia A or B, thalassaemia and von Willebrand disease, as it has a role in determining disease severity.

Allelic genes are said to be **co-dominant** if both alleles are transcribed and translated such that the products of both are found. However, it is often the case that only one allele, the **dominant** allele is expressed, the second, non-expressed allele being termed **recessive**. Thus, a recessive allele will only be expressed in an individual who is homozygous for that recessive allele, i.e. when no dominant allele is present.

An example of co-dominant gene alleles is found in the ABO system, where the AB blood group results from the inheritance of the two co-dominant gene alleles, *A* and *B*, one gene allele originating from the mother and one from the father.

Genotype and phenotype

The terms **genotype** and **phenotype** were described by Johannsen in 1909. **Genotype** can be defined as meaning all or a particular part of the genetic constitution of an individual or a cell. In the transfusion laboratory, the genotype of an individual refers to their genetic constitution in relation to a particular blood group. This is often not detectable by the laboratory but may be surmised by investigating the family or by the use of direct genetic techniques (see Chapter 13). An individual who shows results consistent with blood group A may have the genotype *AA* or *AO* depending on the inheritance of the *A* and *O* alleles from the parents (see *Fig. 4.2*). It may be important to know the *Rh* genotype, for example in the case of the father of a baby at risk of developing haemolytic disease of the newborn (see Chapter 8). **Phenotype** is defined as the observable effects of a gene; thus, the phenotype can be deduced by the results of tests in the laboratory. Blood group B individuals are phenotypically group B, but we cannot tell using laboratory tests based on red cell agglutination whether they carry *BB* or *BO* genes, i.e. what their genotype is. The genotype and phenotype of blood group AB are the same, and this is evident because the products of both genes are expressed. Similarly, blood group O has the same genotype and phenotype, as individuals can only be carrying the *O* allele.

Genes linked to the X chromosome

The genes responsible for particular blood group antigens may be carried on the autosomal chromosomes or, rarely, on the sex chromosomes. When they are carried on the sex chromosomes, they are linked to the X chromosome. The only example of a red cell antigen inherited on the X chromosome is XG^a (incidence of Xg^a = 89% females, 66% males). Another example of X linkage which may be of interest is the inheritance of the defective coagulation disease, haemophilia A, which is briefly described in Chapter 9.

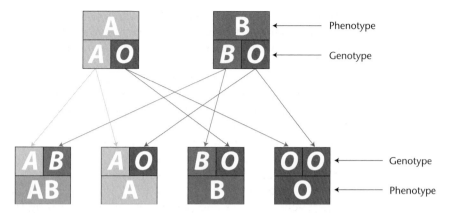

Figure 4.2
Inheritance of phenotypes in the ABO blood group system.

Gene dominance

Genes also may be dominant, co-dominant or recessive; thus, they can be inherited in a variety of ways. However, most blood groups fall into the category of autosomal dominant or co-dominant inheritance, with multiple generations affected, each affected person normally having one affected parent, and with males and females being equally affected.

Patterns of inheritance

Family pedigrees are sometimes used to trace the inheritance of a particular gene. The term **propositus** (or **proposita**) is used to indicate the individual who is carrying the gene of interest. Pedigree charts use specific symbols to describe the family tree in a diagrammatic form as shown in *Fig. 4.3*.

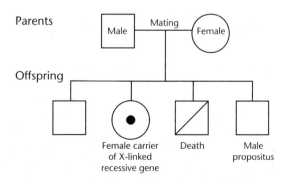

Figure 4.3
Example of a pedigree chart illustrating the symbols used.

Inheritance patterns are also of value when considering population genetics for blood groups, that is, the frequency with which a blood group gene occurs in a given population. See *Box 4.2* for a brief explanation of the Hardy–Weinberg principle.

Box 4.2 Population gene frequencies

The Hardy–Weinberg formula has been used to determine the frequency of a gene in a population. Hardy was a mathematician and Weinberg was a physician who together addressed the possible reason why a recessive trait would not eventually be lost from a population. They produced a mathematical formula, based on the binomial equation, which requires certain conditions for its basis. These include a large population with random mating, no mutations and no migration. Whilst these are not entirely true of the human population, the formula has nevertheless been of use in determining population genetics.

The formula is based on the multiplication of binomials. It can be applied to establish the frequencies of mutant alleles in a given population and relate this to the frequency of allele pairings of homozygotes with the 'normal' allele only, homozygotes with the 'mutant' allele only (known as 'trait' in disorders such as sickle cell disease, though not in blood groups) and heterozygotes, made up of mixed allele pairs who are 'carriers' of the recessive trait or else display the trait if it is dominant.

Statistics of population gene frequencies have been widely used in transfusion science to estimate the most likely genotype for an individual where the results indicate that more than one possibility may exist. This has been useful in the past for determining the multiple alleles of the Rh system and is referred to in more detail in Chapter 6. An awareness of the population frequencies of blood groups is also useful in the screening of compatible blood for transfusion to a patient. If the patient is known to possess a number of different antibodies to blood groups, an increased number of units of donor blood must be screened before compatible blood can be selected.

SUGGESTED FURTHER READING

Campbell, N.A. and Reece, J.B. (2005) *Biology*, 7th edn. San Francisco: Pearson.

Daniels, G. (2002) *Human Blood Groups*. Oxford: Blackwell Science.

Daniels, G. (2004) Molecular blood grouping. *Vox Sanguinis* **87**(Suppl. 1), 563–566.

Read, A.P. and Donnai, D. (2007) *New Clinical Genetics*. Oxford: Scion.

Reid, M.E. and Rios, M. (1999) Applications of molecular genotyping to immunohaematology. *British Journal of Biomedical Science* **56**, 145–152.

The Blood Group Antigen Gene Mutation Database:
http://www.ncbi.nlm.nih.gov/projects/mhc/xslcgi.fcgi?cmd=bgmut/home

SELF-ASSESSMENT QUESTIONS

1. Define the term 'codon'.
2. Define the term 'allele'.
3. List the organic bases of DNA.
4. What type of inheritance would show a gene appearing in each generation with equal frequency between the sexes?
5. Differentiate between independent assortment and dependent assortment of genetic material (genes).
6. What is the role of tRNA in protein synthesis?
7. Describe three types of genetic mutation.
8. Give an example of how nucleotide substitution can affect the production of a blood group antigen.
9. In blood group terms, what are the gene products?

CHAPTER 5

Introduction to blood groups: the ABO system

Learning objectives

After studying this chapter you should be able to:

■ Explain the nomenclature of selected blood groups

■ Describe the nature and functional groups of blood group antigens

■ Discuss the historical aspects of the ABO system

■ Outline the cellular and molecular basis of the ABO system

■ Describe the genetics of the ABO system

■ Describe the frequency of ABO in selected populations

5.1 INTRODUCTION

Red blood cells bear numerous cell surface structures that can be recognized as antigens by the immune system of individuals who lack that particular structure. Recipients of a blood transfusion may produce antibodies to an entire structure, or a single or limited number of epitopes. Similarly, a pregnant woman may produce antibodies to foreign antigens expressed on her foetus' red blood cells. More than 600 antigens have been defined on human red cells. The International Society of Blood Transfusion (ISBT) has tabulated 23 blood group systems and five blood group collections. A blood group system is defined as a cluster of blood group antigens encoded by alternative forms of the same gene. In recent years, the biochemical and molecular bases for many of these antigens have been elucidated, as have the biological roles for many blood group antigen structures. Additionally, associations between some antigenic phenotypes and disease have been identified. The surface components which are responsible for antigen expression may be divided into carbohydrate and protein structures.

The carbohydrate antigens are expressed by immunodominant sugars which are attached to a precursor molecule by the action of glycosyl transferase enzymes. These enzymes are the products of the blood group genes. The carbohydrate structures are attached covalently to glycolipids or glycoproteins and are synthesized in the Golgi apparatus of erythropoietic cells.

The molecular bases of carbohydrate antigens depend on polymorphic variations in the genes which synthesize their glycosyl transferase enzymes, e.g. ABO, Hh, Lewis, P or Ii. Protein antigens are defined by amino acid sequence changes in red cell membrane proteins, which are generated by nucleotide sequence variation at the DNA level. Broadly, they fall into six functional groups:

- membrane transporters or channels, e.g. Rh, Kidd, Diego, Colton, KX
- membrane-bound enzymes, e.g. Kell, Cartwright
- structural or assembly proteins, e.g. MNS, Gerbich
- chemokine receptors, e.g. Duffy
- cell adhesion molecules, e.g. Lutheran, LW, Xg, Indian
- complement regulatory proteins, e.g. Cromer, Knops, Chido/Rodgers

5.2 BLOOD GROUP NOMENCLATURE

Unfortunately, over the years, the naming of blood group antigens has been inconsistent and confusing. Originally, single letters were used to name blood group antigens such as A and B. The symbol O (zero) meant no antigens were present, until, that is, the discovery of H. Single letters continued to be used for the allelic pair M and N, and for P (although now called P_1). This continued with the Rh antigens C, D and E but with the introduction of lower-case letters to describe allelic pairs of antigens, C and c, D and d, E and e. This system was also used for S and s, K and k, and unfortunately also, for I and i, which are not an allelic pair. Where subgroups of antigens were identified, it became common practice to use subscript numbers, e.g. A_1, A_2, P_1, P_2. The discovery of the Lewis system brought a change to using the first two letters of the proposita's surname (Le) with the addition of a superscript letter a for the first antigen of an allelic pair to be recognized, and a superscript letter b for the second. Le^a and Le^b, however, were not found to be the products of allelic genes.

This system worked for Duffy and Kidd but in order to avoid confusion with Rh D, the Duffy antigens were named using the last two letters of the proposita's name (FY). The Kidd antigens were named using the proposita's initials (JK) in order to avoid confusion with K of Kell and Rh D. Similar manipulations of names with superscript letters a, b and most other letters of the alphabet in lower or upper case continue to be used. In the early 1960s, numerical systems were proposed for the antigens of the Kell and Rh systems. Thus, phenotypes could be represented by a series of numbers, positive if the antigen was present and negative if the antigen was absent. For example, in the Rh system, D = 1, C = 2, E = 3, c = 4, e = 5, so that DCce (R_1r) becomes Rh:1,2,–3,4,5. These systems carried no genetic implications and proved to be unwieldy in normal conversation.

In 1980, the ISBT set up a Working Party on Terminology for Red Cell Surface Antigens. The aim was to produce a uniform system of terminology which was both eye-readable and capable of being adapted for computer use, and which was in keeping with the genetic basis of the blood groups. Each known antigen was given a unique six-digit number, the first three numbers indicating the blood group system and the second three the antigen itself. Existing terminologies were retained and system symbols included. For example, the Kell system is 006 and the K antigen 001, so K may be represented as 006001. Alternatively, the system symbol (KEL) may be used so that K may also be represented as KEL001. As it is permissible to omit the leading zeros, it is more common to see K represented as KEL1. In addition to these variations in naming blood group antigens, there have been problems concerning how the antigens, antibodies and genes should appear on the printed page.

The ABO blood groups will be considered in detail in this chapter because of their importance in blood transfusion. Other blood group systems, which will be described in the following chapters, are: Rh, Lewis, P, Ii, Kidd, Kell, Duffy, Lutheran and MNS.

The following convention has been adopted throughout this book:

- existing 'popular' terminology is used for blood systems and antigens
- superscripts and subscripts are used where appropriate
- presence or absence of antigens is indicated with + or − signs respectively
- genes are written in italics
- antibodies are written as their antigen notation, with the prefix anti-
- ISBT notations are also included

The earliest reports of blood transfusions in modern times appeared in the 17th century. One of the first successful transfusions of human blood took place in 1825 when a woman who lost blood in labour was revived by blood donated by her husband. However, blood transfusion was often fatal until the experiments by Landsteiner in 1900 gave evidence of the ABO blood group system.

5.3 THE ABO BLOOD GROUP SYSTEM (ISBT 001, SYMBOL ABO)

The ABO system consists of the blood groups A, B, AB and O, with further subdivisions of A and B. The nomenclature is based on the presence of oligosaccharides, which act as blood group antigens due to their ability to bind to antibodies. These antigens can be detected on red blood cells, white blood cells, platelets, endothelial cells lining blood vessels and many other body cells. They are also present in body fluids, provided the individual has the required gene. Testing of blood for transfusion to determine the ABO group is imperative in order to prevent blood transfusion reactions, the result of which may be fatal.

Landsteiner discovered three of the four blood groups in the ABO system in 1900. This was also the year in which Gregor Mendel's laws of heredity were rediscovered, having first been proposed in 1895. The subsequent discoveries in blood groups allowed for much progress in genetic knowledge. Karl Landsteiner was a remote, austere man who was awarded the Nobel prize in medicine in 1930 for his discovery of blood groups. He was a well-trained scientist and knew the value of controls. The use of controls in the finding of red cell 'agglutinogens' and serum 'agglutinins' led to Landsteiner's discovery of the ABO system. Landsteiner was working at the Institute of Pathological Anatomy in Vienna, Austria, in 1900 when he conducted his experiment on six men from his laboratory. These included four researchers, an unknown man labelled 'Zar' and Karl Landsteiner himself. Blood was taken from each and separated into cells and serum by allowing it to clot. The red cells were diluted in saline to a suspension of 5% concentration and each serum placed in a test tube with each sample of red cells. This gave 36 results which could either show agglutination or remain unagglutinated. The red cells of two samples, Landsteiner and another colleague, showed no agglutination with any of the other sera, but their sera did agglutinate the red cells of the other four. The results of the other four samples fell into two groups of two, each showing reciprocal agglutination patterns. It was also noted that no cell sample was agglutinated by its own serum. The two patterns of agglutination were called 'A' and 'B', respectively, and the serum with both agglutinins was initially called 'C', then later 'O' (for zero reaction). Thus, the ABO system was first described. It is interesting to note, considering the frequency of occurrence of the ABO groups in the German population at the time, that the chance of Landsteiner testing six men at random and finding two of each blood group – A, B and O – is 0.031! However, Landsteiner was to become the founder of immunochemistry and immunohaematology.

'Landsteiner's law' states that the presence of the antigen on the cells implies the absence of the corresponding antibody in the serum and the presence of the opposite antibody. Thus, group O individuals would have antibodies to both A and B antigen. A fourth blood group in which both antigens were detectable was described in 1902 by von DeCastello and Sturli. This was called AB and neither antibody A nor B could be detected in the serum of these individuals. *Table 5.1* shows the antigens and antibodies of the ABO system and *Table 5.2* shows the results of ABO blood grouping using known antisera and red blood cells.

Gel cards for groups O (Rh + and –), A, B and AB are given in *Colour plate 1*.

Table 5.1 The red cell antigens and serum antibodies of the ABO system

Red cell antigens	Serum antibodies	Blood group
Antigen A	Antibody B	A
Antigen B	Antibody A	B
Neither A nor B	Antibodies A and B	O
Both A and B	Neither A nor B antibodies	AB

N.B. The blood group is always designated by the antigens on the red cells. The antigens are detectable on foetal red blood cells and throughout life.

Table 5.2 Results of ABO blood grouping using known antisera and red cells

Red cell sample

Patient	Agglutination		Blood group
	using anti-A	using anti-B	
1	+	–	A
2	–	+	B
3	+	+	AB
4	–	–	O

Serum sample

Patient	Agglutination		Blood group
	using A cells	using B cells	
1	–	+	A
2	+	–	B
3	–	–	AB
4	+	+	O

5.4 THE BIOCHEMICAL NATURE OF THE A AND B ANTIGENS

Molecular biology techniques have made it possible to classify blood group antigens into categories which relate to cellular function, such as transporters and channels, adhesion molecules, receptors and ligands, and enzymes and structural proteins. Thus, the structures of the enzymes for the ABO blood group have been established during the 1990s. The ABO blood group is really a histo-blood group system due to its antigens being expressed on most tissues and secreted in body fluids. The A and B antigens are defined by specific **sugars** attached to a chain of **oligosaccharides** which protrude from the red cell membrane. An understanding of red cell membrane structure is helpful and you are advised to look carefully at *Fig. 5.1*. The 'precursor chain', as the remainder of the oligosaccharide chain is known, is attached to **glyco-lipids**, which form part of the red blood cell membrane structure and which have a role in the transport of anions and glucose across the membrane. Before the sugars for the A and B antigens can be attached to the precursor chain, it is necessary that the individual is genetically able to attach L-**fucose**, which is known as the **H antigen**, to this chain of molecules. Oligosaccharides are carbohydrate polymers of between 3 and 20 sugar residues. They attach by covalent bonds to lipid and protein, often forming a branched structure of side chains, which allows for a great variety of shapes and sizes due to the many possibilities for linking within the chains. This results in a large number of different blood groups as each configuration appears different and evokes an antibody-producing response in a person not

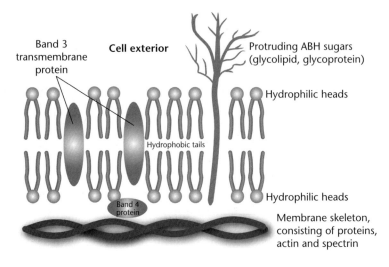

Figure 5.1
Diagrammatic structure of the red cell membrane.

already carrying that 'antigen' on their red blood cells. Other biochemical sugars which are important in blood group antigen structures are ceramides, which are fatty acids joined to sphingosine by an amide linkage, and gangliosides. Gangliosides differ from cerebrosides in that their oligosaccharide head group contains one to four **sialic acid** residues which are negatively charged at pH 7, giving the red cell surface an overall negative charge.

The sugars involved in the ABO system are L-fucose, *N*-acetyl-galactosamine (the 'A' antigen) and D-galactose (the 'B' antigen). It is the specificity of the sugars present on the red cell which makes the ABO groups antigenic when transfused to individuals who lack those antigens.

The blood group-determining sugars are added to the red cell membrane in the Golgi apparatus of the cells. Enzymes are required for the attachment

---

Box 5.1 The effects of coffee beans

Group O blood is the only safe option if there is any doubt about the recipient's blood group, as well as being the most common, and therefore it is in high demand. However, in the 1980s an enzyme from green coffee beans was shown to remove the B antigen from red blood cells. Henrik Clausen at the University of Copenhagen in Denmark and his colleagues have continued this research and discovered more powerful enzymes in bacteria and fungi. Two enzymes have been reported in 2007 to be of use. One, from a gut bacterium called *Bacteroides fragilis*, has the ability to remove the B antigen. The other, from *Elizabethkingia meningoseptica*, a cause of opportunistic infections, removes the A antigen. The researchers found that the *B. fragilis* enzyme is used up a thousand times more slowly than the coffee bean enzyme. Clinical trials are needed to test whether the treated blood is safe and effective.

of the sugars to the pre-existing chain of molecules. These enzymes are glycosyl transferases and their role is to transfer sugar molecules. The production of these transferases is dependent on the presence of the gene specific for their formation.

5.5   GENES INVOLVED IN THE ABO SYSTEM

The use of molecular techniques in the last decade or so has provided a wealth of information to identify and classify the alleles of the ABO system. We are now aware of the variety and complexity of types and subtypes of blood groups caused by mutations, deletions and substitutions of nucleotides within gene alleles. As research continues, the student should note that this is both a fascinating and growing body of knowledge.

The molecular basis of ABO blood group expression was established using cDNA cloning of the glycosyl transferase for blood group A in 1990 by Yamamoto *et al.* The *ABO* gene responsible for the enzyme production has been located on chromosome 9. It consists of seven exons and the alleles for *A1* and *B* differ in exons 6 and 7. This results in a difference of seven nucleotides which encode four amino acids. These four amino acids are substituted at positions 176, 235, 266 and 268 and the resulting glycosyl transferases therefore differ by four amino acids (see *Table 5.3*).

Table 5.3   Amino acid substitutions in glycosyltranferases of blood groups A and B

Amino acid position	Amino acid (A)	Amino acid (B)
176	Arginine	Glycine
235	Glycine	Serine
266	Leucine	Methionine
268	Glycine	Alanine

The *FUT1(H)* gene encodes the enzyme **α1,2-fucosyl transferase**, which transfers the sugar L-fucose (Fuc) to the terminal sugar of the membrane chain, galactose. This is known as the **H** antigen and is the structure found in individuals of the blood group O, as well as being a necessary precursor for the addition of the A and B antigens. It is now known that there are two genes regulating the production of H antigen: *FUT1* is responsible for its presence on red cells and *FUT2* is responsible for H in other tissues and body fluids.

If an individual is homozygous for mutations in the *FUT1(H)* gene which make it inactive, then no H antigen is produced (a rare occurrence). The absence of H, that is no L-fucose attached, means that neither A nor B sugars can attach to the membrane chain. So, despite the genes for A or B being present, the individual is unable to attach the A- or B-determining sugars and thus they appear to be blood group O when tested by agglutination techniques.

The *A* allele encodes **N-acetyl-galactosaminyl transferase**, which transfers *N*-acetyl-galactosamine (GalNAc) to the H structure, giving the A antigen that is found on the red cells of blood group A individuals. The *B* allele encodes **D-galactosyl transferase**, which transfers D-galactose (Gal) to the H structure, resulting in blood group B. However, if both *A* and *B* alleles are present on the chromosome, both sugars are attached to the H structure in a random way as is found on the red cells of blood group AB individ-

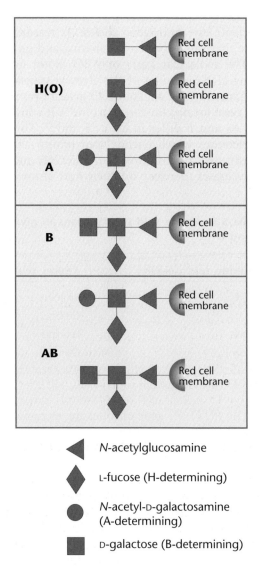

N-acetylglucosamine

L-fucose (H-determining)

N-acetyl-D-galactosamine (A-determining)

D-galactose (B-determining)

Figure 5.2
Biochemical basis of the ABO blood group system.

uals. The nature and sequence of the sugars and the type of glycosidic bond joining the sugars together are important in conferring antigenicity. The precursor chain of molecules may be formed by linkage of the sugars to each other at different positions. Type 1 chains exhibit α1–3 linkage in which the carbon at position 1 of galactose is attached to the carbon at position 3 of *N*-acetyl-glucosamine in the precursor sugar. Type 2 chains show a β1–4 linkage. L-fucose is attached to the precursor chain of molecules by α1–2 linkage. *Fig. 5.2* shows the biochemical basis of the structures of the A, B and H antigens, illustrating the sugars involved and the way in which they are attached to each other resulting in a tetrasaccharide structure.

5.6 SECRETORS OF A, B AND H SUGARS

The A, B and H sugars may also be secreted into the body fluids such as plasma, sweat, saliva, semen, breast milk, tears and digestive juices, with the exception of cerebrospinal fluid due to the blood–brain barrier. They are widely distributed on a range of cells including white blood cells (leucocytes), platelets, epithelial cells, spermatozoa and gastric mucosal cells. In embryonic development, these are all cells derived from the endoderm.

In order that the sugars may be secreted, the individual must carry the gene which confers 'secretor status', the *FUT2(Se)* gene. Thus, endodermically derived tissues have H antigen generated by α1,2-L-fucosyl transferase. This enzyme acts on the terminal galactose of the type 1 precursor chain (the secreted ABH glycoprotein sugars are attached by both type 1 and 2 linkage, whereas the ABH sugars are attached by type 1 linkage only). About 20% of the population lack the *FUT2(Se)* gene and are non-secretors and thus have little or no expression of ABO sugars in body fluids, although they may be present on red cells as antigens. The ability to secrete A, B and H sugars may be inherited in the homozygous or heterozygous state. Approximately 80% of the Caucasian population are secretors of the ABH blood group sugars. The ability to secrete ABH sugars into body fluids can be detected by testing the saliva for the presence of A, B or H sugars. Thus, blood group A individuals will secrete A and H sugars, group B will have B and H sugars, and AB individuals will have A, B and H sugars in their saliva. Group O individuals secrete only H sugar.

5.7 THE *FUT1 (H)* GENE AND THE BOMBAY BLOOD GROUPS

The presence and importance of the gene for H antigen was demonstrated by a family study described by Bhende in 1952. This study showed that the presence of the gene, inherited either as the homozygous or heterozygous form, is necessary for the transfer of the A- and/or B-determining oligosaccharide precursor sugar onto the L-fucose of the precursor chain. Thus, individuals whose *FUT1 (H)* gene is inactive (due to mutations) are unable to attach A and B antigens (i.e. sugars) to the red cell membrane, even though they possess the *ABO* gene. Consequently, when these individuals are tested in the laboratory, their red blood cells give the agglutination reaction of group O although their serum contains the antibodies anti-A, anti-B and anti-H. This is known as a 'Bombay blood group' and individuals are denoted as being blood group O_hA, O_hB or O_h. Whilst this is a rare blood group, it is important to detect this blood type in the laboratory, as blood from a Bombay phenotype is not compatible with other ABO groups and such an individual needs to be transfused with Bombay-type blood. The case study in *Box 5.2* describes an example of a Bombay blood group.

Box 5.2 Bombay blood type and haemolytic disease of the newborn

The following case study describes a conundrum surrounding a young Pakistani lady who became pregnant for the second time. The babies were born without any problems despite the mother having been tested as Bombay blood group O_h. This blood type is very rare and has a frequency of approximately 1 in 7600 in India. Her serum was found to contain a strong antibody capable of haemolysing red cells known as anti-H. Her husband tested positive for the H antigen, so the infants should have been positive for H antigen also. This would mean that they should have suffered with haemolytic disease of the newborn due to the strong maternal antibody produced in response to their H antigen. In fact, the babies were both born well and healthy and did not require any blood transfusions for haemolysis. Because Bombay blood group O_h is so rare, some of this blood type was put on standby by the blood centre in case it was needed. It is a mystery why they were not affected by the antibody. It is apparent that they were heterozygous for the H antigen, and when the anti-H antibody crossed the placenta it was 'used up' or 'absorbed' by other tissues expressing H antigen. (Taken from a report by Bhattacharya *et al.,* 2002.)

5.8 INHERITANCE AND MOLECULAR GENETICS OF THE ABO GROUPS

The phenotype is the detectable blood group and the genotype refers to the genetic information upon which the phenotype is based (see Chapter 4). Each individual inherits two genes, one from each parent; thus, the genotypes may be either *AA, AO, BB, BO, AB* or *OO*. The difference between A_1 and A_2 antigens is due to the quantity of antigenic sites and to differences in the antigens themselves. The four alleles could give rise to six possible phenotypes: A_1, A_2, B, O, A_1B or A_2B. The *A* and *B* alleles are co-dominant so that they are expressed if they are present on the chromosome.

Blood group O phenotypes are a result of three different alleles. The prototype allele, O^1, is the most common. It is due to a single base deletion of codon 87 in exon 6 of the *ABO* gene. This causes a **frameshift mutation**, the result of which is that an inactive polypeptide chain consisting of 117 amino acids is produced. In other words, there is a shift in the reading frame, introducing a translation stop codon before the region in which the catalytic enzyme site is produced. Thus, the polypeptide chain produced has no enzyme activity and so is unable to transfer A or B sugars to the red cell membrane. It is thought that 56% of blood group O individuals belong to this type. The second allele for blood group O is found in 40% of the

Table 5.4 ABO phenotypes and genotypes

Phenotype	Possible genotype
A_1	A_1A_1 or A_1A_2 or A_1O
A_2	A_2A_2 or A_2O
B	BB or BO
O	OO
A_1B	A_1B
A_2B	A_2B

population and is known as the O^{lv} type. This also has the same base deletion but in addition there are at least nine nucleotide substitutions in the *ABO* gene. A rare allele (approximately 4% of the population), designated O^2, is due to a **missense mutation** resulting in an enzymatically inactive transferase.

Table 5.4 illustrates the phenotypes and genotypes of the ABO blood group system.

5.9 SUBGROUPS OF A AND B BLOOD GROUPS

Variations in the number of A or B antigen sites on the membrane of the red blood cell have led to the establishment of subgroups. The A antigen has been found to exist in two main subgroups and a number of minor subgroups. The majority of individuals who group as A are those with red blood cells expressing both A_1 and A antigens, and are thus termed blood group A_1; those with only the one form of A antigen are typed as A_2. The presence of A_1 and A_2 subgroups is based on the expression of enzymes (*N*-acetyl-galactosaminyl transferases) which possess different kinetic properties, due to either substitutions or deletions of the allelic residues and an extended reading frame. The resulting transferase is less efficient. This results in some blood group A types expressing less A antigen than others. The presence of the A_1 antigen on red cells can be detected using a **plant lectin** specific to the A_1 antigen. This has been extracted from the seeds of the plant *Dolichos biflorus* and is available commercially. Red cells which test positive with the lectin are typed as A_1. Subgroup A_2 individuals show a weak agglutination when incubated with anti-A. Subgroups A_3 and A_x have much less A antigen present on the cells, sometimes called diminished expression. Other weak subgroups are A_m and A_{el}. The latter has an absence of transferase activity. The A_1A_1 genotype appears as A_1 because of the masking effect of the A_1 gene, i.e it produces both A_1 and A antigen – the latter is indistinguishable from the A antigen produced by the A_2 gene.

Blood group B also contains some weaker forms identified as B_3, B_x and B_m, which are rarely seen in Caucasian populations, although they may be slightly more frequent in Indian, black and oriental populations, each of which have a higher incidence of blood group B.

5.10   POPULATION DISTRIBUTION OF ABO GROUPS

The ABO blood groups are distributed differently in various populations and this may be determined by inheritance and population mobility. It is generally accepted that blood group O is the most common throughout the UK, but there are regional differences, e.g. blood group A was found to be most frequent in northwest England transfusion centres. The population of the USA may be broadly considered in terms of Western European descent, in which 'A' is the most common (45%) followed by 'O' (43%), and African descent, in which 50% of the population are blood group 'O', 29% are 'A' and 17% are group 'B'. In each case, group AB is rare, with approximately 4% incidence. Thus, the distribution of ABO phenotypes varies in different populations throughout the world (see *Table 5.5*).

Table 5.5   Distribution of ABO phenotypes in various populations (%)

Phenotype	Caucasian	Black	Oriental	Indian	Australian aborigine	Native American
O	44	49	43	31	44	100
A$_1$	33	19	27	26	56	0
A$_2$	10	8	rare	3	0	0
B	9	20	25	30	0	0
A$_1$B	3	3	5	9	0	0
A$_2$B	1	1	rare	1	0	0

Box 5.3   A case of acquired B blood group in a previously group A individual

Some enzymes have been found in bacteria which have the ability to 'deacetylate' the carbohydrate structures which make up the A antigen. These enzymes remove the *N*-acetylgalactosamine, and produce galactosamine which has a similar structure to galactose, the sugar for the B antigen. Rare cases of *Escherichia coli* infection have been reported to affect patients in this way; thus, it appears that their blood group has changed from A to B! In addition, this phenomenon is sometimes seen in patients with bowel cancer.

5.11   THE DISTRIBUTION OF ABO-DETERMINING ANTIGENS

The number of antigens, known as the antigenic density, varies among different ABO groups and at different stages of the red blood cell development as the cell membrane is becoming established. Also, the cells obtainable from the umbilical cord of a newborn infant have significantly fewer antigen sites for A, B and H expressed on their surface than the red cells from an adult. It is important to be aware of this in the laboratory detection of blood groups as fewer antigen sites results in a weaker agglutination reaction. The number of antigens gradually increases from foetal life until adolescence. A comparison of antigen site numbers can be seen in *Table 5.6.*

Table 5.6 Number of A, B and H antigens on red blood cells

Cell type	Antigen	Number of antigen sites per cell
A_1 adult	A	800 000–1 000 000
A_2 adult	A	250 000
A_3 adult	A	35 000
A_4 adult	A	4800
A_1 cord	A	250 000–300 000
A_1B adult	A	460 000–850 000
A_2B adult	A	140 000
B adult	B	750 000
B cord	B	200 000–300 000
A_1B adult	B	430 000
O adult	H	1 700 000
O cord	H	325 000
AB cord	H	70 000

5.12 ABO BLOOD GROUP ANTIBODIES

ABO blood group antibodies are present in the sera of healthy adults and older children. The antibodies are formed when the corresponding antigen is absent, a phenomenon sometimes known as 'Landsteiner's law'. Thus, antibody A (anti-A) is found in the sera of groups B and O and anti-B is found in groups A and O. If both A and B antigens are present on the red cells, as in group AB, no antibodies are formed and if neither A nor B antigens are present, as in group O, both anti-A and anti-B are formed. Anti-A_1 is found in the sera of groups B and O as a component of anti-A, i.e the anti-A produced is a mixture of anti-A and anti-A_1. Also found in the sera of group A_1, A_1B and B adults is anti-H. Anti-H is always found in the sera of individuals who carry the rare Bombay blood type.

The antibodies are usually of the IgM class, although they may occur as a mixture of IgM, IgG and Ig A. They are formed at 3–6 months of age, gradually increasing in strength to peak at age 5–10 years. Although they are called 'naturally occurring' antibodies, they result from the stimulus of non-pathogenic microorganisms associated with ingested food. The antibodies react optimally with their corresponding antigens at room temperature, approximately 16–22°C. Thus, they are considered to be 'cold agglutinating antibodies'. They also are able to bind complement at 37°C and in this event would be of concern when transfused to a patient. In addition, anti-A and anti-B may occur as immune, IgG antibodies if their production is stimulated by pregnancy or blood transfusion. These antibodies readily cross the placenta and may cause haemolytic disease of the newborn. Thus, they are considered to be the most clinically significant of all the blood group antibodies. A transfusion of ABO-incompatible blood, meaning the transfusion of group A blood to group O or group B patients, or group B blood to group O or A patients, is often fatal. Blood group O is sometimes transfused in emergencies to patients who are group A or B. This may also be fatal if the donor blood contains a high titre of anti-A or anti-B haemolysins (i.e. antibodies which cause haemolysis of red cells). Immune anti-A and anti-B may also cause haemolytic disease of the newborn although this is rare and usually mild. See Chapter 8 for more information on haemolytic disease of the newborn.

SUGGESTED FURTHER READING

Avent, N. (1996) Human erythrocyte antigen expression: its molecular bases. *British Journal of Biomedical Science* **54**, 16–37.

Bhattacharya, S., Makar, Y., Laycock, R.A., Poole, J. and Hadley, A. (2002) Outcome of consecutive pregnancies in a patient with Bombay (O$_h$) blood group. *Transfusion Medicine* **12**, 379–381.

Daniels, G.L., Poole, J., de Silva, M, Callaghan, T., MacLennan, S. and Smith, N. (2002) The clinical significance of blood group antibodies. *Transfusion Medicine* **12**, 287–295.

Murphy, M.F. and Pamphilon, D.H. (eds) (2005) *Practical Transfusion Medicine*, 2nd edn. Oxford: Blackwell Publishing.

Watkins, W.M. (2001) Commemoration of the centenary of the discovery of the ABO blood group system. *Transfusion Medicine* **11**, 239–351.

Yamamoto, F. (2000) Molecular genetics of ABO. *Vox Sanguinis* **78**, 91–103.

SELF-ASSESSMENT QUESTIONS

1. What is the structure of the *ABO* gene?
2. Name the enzymes produced in blood groups A, B and O, respectively.
3. Which sugar must be attached to the precursor oligosaccharide chain on the red cell in all ABO groups?
4. Compare the effects on an individual of an absence of the *FUT1* gene with absence of the *FUT2* gene.
5. Name the immunodominant sugars for the blood groups A, B and O.
6. Compare the frequency of ABO groups in Caucasian, Black and Indian populations.
7. Draw a table showing the naturally occurring antibodies present in blood groups A, B, AB and O.
8. What is the defect which results in subgroups of blood group A?
9. At what temperature do antibodies A and B optimally agglutinate red cells?

Introduction to the Rh blood group system

Learning objectives
After studying this chapter you should be able to:

■ Discuss the historical aspects of the Rh systems

■ Outline the cellular and molecular bases of the Rh systems

■ Describe the genetics of the Rh systems

■ Describe the frequency of Rh types in different populations

■ Discuss the contribution of molecular techniques to knowledge of the Rh blood group systems

6.1 INTRODUCTION TO THE RH SYSTEM (ISBT 004, SYMBOL RH)

The Rh system was discovered in 1940 by Landsteiner and Wiener. They injected rabbits and guinea pigs with the red cells from *Macacus rhesus* monkeys and the resulting antibody reacted with the red cells of 85% of New York blood donors. Those who reacted were said to have the Rhesus factor and were Rhesus positive, whilst those that did not react lacked the Rhesus factor and were Rhesus negative. The terms Rhesus positive, or Rh positive, and Rhesus negative, or Rh negative, are still used (incorrectly) today, especially by clinical staff, to describe what we now know as Rh D positive and Rh D negative.

In 1939, Levine and Stetson had described an antibody in a mother who had recently had a stillborn foetus. The antibody caused a haemolytic transfusion reaction when she was transfused with ABO-compatible blood from her husband. They suggested that the antibody had been produced in response to an antigen carried by the foetus, which had been inherited from the father. This antibody was subsequently shown to have the same reaction pattern as Landsteiner and Wiener's anti-Rh, and so Rh haemolytic disease of the newborn was described for the first time.

By 1945, the original Rh factor had been renamed D and four more Rh antigens discovered. These were the antithetical antigens C and c, and E and e (for further information about antithetical genes, see Chapter 4). There

---

Box 6.1   Numerical system for Rh

In 1962, Rosenfield and colleagues proposed a numerical system for describing the Rh antigens. This system was free from the genetic implications of either Wiener's or Fisher's systems, as it merely recorded the observed serological reactions. The known Rh antigens were numbered from 1 (for D) to 24, in order of discovery. The numbering of Rh antigens has now reached 52, although, because of obsolete forms, there are now 45 antigens in the system.

---

are now 45 antigens (see *Box 6.1*) in the Rh system but D, C, c, E and e are the most commonly identified and the most significant in blood transfusion. The Rh antigens are expressed on polypeptides. The Rh polypeptides span the red cell membrane exposing six extracellular loops on which are expressed the Rh antigens. These polypeptides are associated in the membrane with an Rh glycoprotein to form tetramers (two Rh polypeptides and two Rh glycoproteins), which form the Rh core complex. The Rh glycoprotein is essential for the formation of this Rh core complex. Mutations in the genes controlling the expression of the Rh polypeptides or the Rh glycoproteins can result in the Rh_{null} phenotype, in which no Rh antigens are expressed. Red cell defects seen in the Rh_{null} phenotype include abnormal cation transport across the red cell membrane and red cell morphological abnormalities, in the form of stomatocytes (red blood cells that exhibit a slit or mouth-shaped pallor rather than a central pallor), which may cause a mild, compensated haemolytic anaemia (see *Fig. 6.1*). The function of the Rh polypeptide is not known for certain, but it seems likely that it is involved in cation transport across the red cell membrane. The Rh antigens are well developed before birth, being detectable in the 6-week-old foetus. They are fully expressed on cord red blood cells. Rh antigens have not been demonstrated on leucocytes and platelets, or found in saliva or amniotic fluid.

The Rh antigens are distributed with considerable variation in different populations. This is illustrated in *Table 6.1*, which shows examples of the variation in distribution of the D antigen.

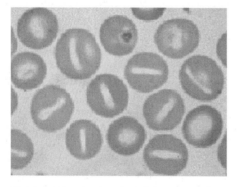

Figure 6.1
Stomatocytes in peripheral blood.

Table 6.1 Examples of the frequency of the D antigen in various populations

	Rh D	
	positive (%)	negative (%)
Europe	83	17
West Africa	97	3
India	90	10
Japan	99.7	0.3
China	93	7

6.2 INHERITANCE AND NOMENCLATURE OF THE RH SYSTEM

Two genetic systems were originally proposed to explain the relationships and inheritance of these five original Rh antigens. In the USA, Wiener proposed a system comprising a single locus producing factors he called agglutinogens, which could express multiple antigens. In the UK, Fisher and Race proposed a system of three closely linked loci for D/d, C/c and E/e, each gene coding for the production of a single antigen. Thus, the antigens C and c were thought to be the products of the co-dominant alleles *C* and *c*. Antigens E and e were thought to be the products of the co-dominant alleles *E* and *e*. The D antigen was the product of the D gene and the proposed allelic gene *d* was considered an amorph as no d antigen or anti-d antibody was ever discovered. Fisher also postulated that the order of the genes on a chromosome was DCE (see *Box 6.2*). It has become common practice to refer to them in this order.

Box 6.2 Fisher's DCE theory

Race and Sanger showed their early Rh typing results to Fisher, in the Bun Shop (a Cambridge pub). His first outline of his DCE theory, on 22 June 1944, was described on a pub beer mat.

The clinical significance of the Rh system has led to considerable investigation of the system. As new Rh antigens and phenotypes were discovered, it became apparent that neither Wiener's nor Fisher's system could explain every new finding. However, Fisher's system of three closely linked loci was the most complete and allowed the deduction of phenotypes of offspring from different mating types. Fisher's shorthand notation was also very convenient for communicating information regarding phenotypes and genotypes.

It has now been shown by modern molecular biology techniques that neither of these earlier systems was completely correct and that in fact the

Table 6.2 Fisher's model of haplotypes and their frequency in the Caucasian population

Haplotype	Shorthand notation	Approx. frequency in Caucasians (%)	Haplotype	Shorthand notation	Approx. frequency in Caucasians (%)
DCe	R_1	41	dCe	r′	1
DcE	R_2	14	dcE	r″	1
Dce	R_0	3	dce	r	39
DCE	R_z	<1	dCE	r^Y	<1
Rh D positive			Rh D negative		

Rh system is controlled by two closely linked loci. One carries the gene for the Rh D polypeptide and is known as the *RHD* locus. The other carries the genes for the CcEe polypeptide and is known as the *RHCE* locus.

Despite current evidence concerning the genetics and biochemistry of the Rh system, Fisher's model and shorthand notation continue to be a convenient way to explain and communicate Rh phenotypes and genotypes. For this reason, it is outlined below in more detail

6.3 FISHER'S DCE SYSTEM

The Fisher model proposed that three pairs of closely linked genes (now known to be two genes) allow for eight possible haplotype arrangements of Rh genes on a chromosome. This is shown in *Table 6.2* and *Fig. 6.2*, and the possible genotypes are shown in *Table 6.3*.

The three genes of each set were thought to be inherited together due to the close linkage of the loci. Each could then be paired with itself or any other arrangement, giving 36 possible genotypes. The eight most common ones are listed in *Table 6.2* with their frequencies.

It should be noted that the vast majority of Rh D-negative individuals are dce/dce (rr) and therefore capable of being immunized by exposure to C+ and E+ red cells.

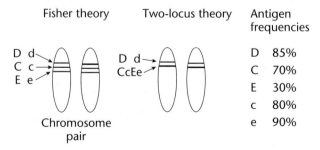

Figure 6.2
Suggested gene locations for the Fisher and two-locus theories.

Table 6.3 Fisher's model of genotypes and their frequency in the Caucasian population

Genotype	Shorthand notation	Approx. frequency (%)	Genotype	Shorthand notation	Approx. frequency (%)
DCe/dce	R_1r	33	*dce/dce*	rr	15
DcE/dce	R_2r	11			
Dce/dce	R_0r	2			
DCe/DCe	R_1R_1	18			
DcE/DcE	R_2R_2	2			
DCe/DcE	R_1R_2	14			
DCe/Dce	R_1R_0	2			
All other combinations		<1	All other combinations		<1
Rh D positive			Rh D negative		

Although current knowledge of the Rh genes has rendered the Fisher model obsolete, it is vital that students are familiar with the Fisher shorthand notations and their implied genotypes. It is with these shorthand expressions that Blood Transfusion Laboratory workers in the UK communicate information on the Rh system on a day-to-day basis.

6.4 THE TWO-LOCUS MODEL

In this model, suggested by Tippett in 1986, the Rh system is controlled by two closely linked loci, *RHD* and *RHCE*. The *RHD* locus carries the gene for the RHD polypeptide, which expresses all the D antigen epitopes. The *RHCE* locus carries the genes for the RHCE polypeptide, which expresses both the C/c and E/e antigens. The genes which encode the C/c and E/e antigens are co-dominant alleles. *RHCE* exists in four allelic forms and each allele determines the expression of two antigens in Ce, ce, cE or CE combination (*RHCE* is the collective name of the four alleles). The Rh genes are located on chromosome 1. *Figs 6.3* and *6.4* are diagrammatic representations of the *RHD* and *RHCE* genes and Rh D-positive and Rh D-negative gene arrangements. *Fig. 6.5* shows the relationship between the two-locus haplotypes and the corresponding Fisher DCE notations.

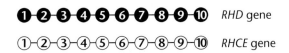

Figure 6.3
Representation of the *RHD* and *RHCE* genes. Each gene contains ten exons, which are shown numbered 1 to 10.

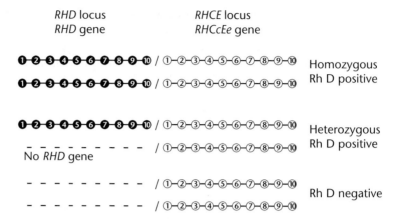

Figure 6.4
Representation of Rh D-positive and Rh D-negative gene arrangements.

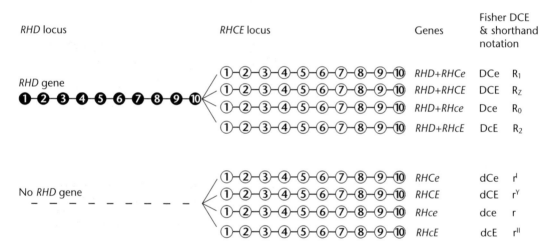

Figure 6.5
Relationship between two-locus haplotypes and Fisher DCE notation.

The *RHD* and *RHCE* loci are very similar, each comprising ten exons. The corresponding polypeptides are therefore very similar, differing only at 36 of the 417 amino acid residues in each polypeptide. The C/c antigen polymorphism appears to be associated with four amino acid substitutions, whereas the E/e polymorphism is associated with a single amino acid substitution (see *Table 6.4*). Transfer of exons between *RHD* and *RHCE* loci, and *vice versa*, is known to occur. This causes variations in epitope expression and hence antigen expression. The location of the RHD and RHCE polypeptide chains in the red cell membrane are depicted in *Figs 6.6* and *6.7*. It can be seen that they are transmembrane proteins.

Table 6.4 Amino acids (AA) involved in the C/c and E/e polymorphisms

Antigen expressed		AA position	Exon
C	c		
cysteine	tryptophan	16	1
isoleucine	leucine	60	2
serine	asparagine	68	2
serine	proline	103*	2
E	e		
proline	alanine	226	5

*This amino acid is located on the second external loop and considered crucial for C/c expression.

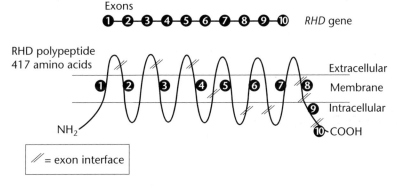

Figure 6.6
RHD polypeptide chain within the red cell membrane. The RHD polypeptide chain is a transmembrane protein which spans the red cell membrane and frequently protrudes on both intra- and extracellular surfaces. Both the NH₂ and COOH termini are located intracellularly. The interface between each of the ten exons and the amino acid point is shown.

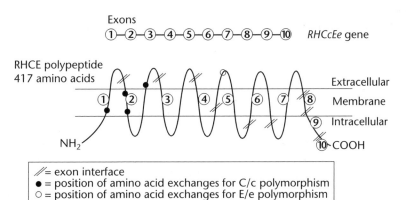

Figure 6.7
RHCE polypeptide.

Expression of Rh epitopes is dependent on the sequence and resulting conformation of the amino acids within the polypeptide chain. Changes in amino acid sequences or exchange of exons can not only lead to the expression of new epitopes, but also cause conformational changes which may affect the expression of other epitopes.

Epitopes are the sites that are recognized by antibodies and thus each antibody has a specific epitope to which it can bind (see Chapter 2). Polyclonal antibodies produced in humans are usually a mixture of antibodies to several related epitopes or groups of epitopes. Monoclonal antibodies, which are used in laboratory testing for Rh status, are more usually specific for a single epitope or group of epitopes (see Chapter 2). The RHD and RHCE polypeptides may be thought of as expressing many different epitopes which together express the antigens of the Rh system.

6.5 QUALITATIVE DIFFERENCES IN RH ANTIGENS

The Rh D antigen is now considered to contain at least 30 different epitopes, as revealed by tests using monoclonal antibodies. Rare individuals who lack certain epitopes are known as **partial D** and may be stimulated to produce antibodies to the missing epitopes by transfusion or pregnancy. The partial D type known as category D^{VI} is the clinically most important partial D (see *Box 6.3* for an explanation of the development of the nomenclature systems for partial D types). Severe cases of haemolytic disease of the newborn have occurred in Rh D-positive babies born to category D^{VI} mothers with anti-D antibody. Category D^{VI} is the most common partial D occurring in 6–10% of weak D samples and 0.02–0.05% of all Caucasian samples. The majority of Rh D-positive individuals with allo-anti-D are category D^{VI}.

This partial D state may arise from the replacement of an exon segment from *RHD* by an equivalent segment from *RHCE*, creating a hybrid *RHD–CE–D* gene (see *Fig. 6.8*) or as a result of point mutation within *RHD*. The replacement of several exon segments from *RHD* with the equivalent segments from *RHCE* can destroy the ability to produce D antigen altogether. Thus, the individual only expresses the C/c and E/e antigens and serologically appears as Rh D negative although they do possess an *RHD* gene.

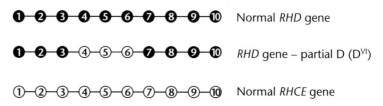

Figure 6.8
This shows how exon exchange gives rise to a partial D gene. Exons 4, 5 and 6 of the *RHD* gene have been replaced with copies of exons 4, 5 and 6 from the *RHCE* gene. This results in the production of an RHD polypeptide which does not express all the normal D epitopes, that is, a partial D.

Box 6.3 The D antigen mosaic

In 1953, Wiener proposed that the Rh D antigen was a mosaic of four parts, which he termed Rh^A, Rh^B, Rh^C and Rh^D. Rare individuals who lack part of this mosaic (partial D) may produce immune anti-D antibody specific for the epitopes they lack. In the 1960s, Tippett identified seven D categories by cross-testing the cells and sera of Rh D-positive individuals with anti-D in their serum. These D categories were designated using superscript Roman numerals I to VII, e.g. category D^{III}, category D^{VI}. Some of the categories were also subdivided. Further partial D types have been identified by their reaction patterns with monoclonal anti-D. There has been no clear systematic approach to naming these partial D types. By 1993, there was a nine-epitope model for Rh D and by 1995 a 30-epitope model. It is now most usual to see partial D types written as their D category (or name if not in a category) together with the epitopes they express and/or lack in either the nine- or 30-epitope models or both. This can make for difficult reading for students, and for even more difficult conversation.

The G antigen

The G antigen is usually only detected on red cells expressing D antigen or C antigen or both. Its expression appears to be dependent on amino acid sequences derived from exon 2 of the *RHD* gene. Anti-G has been implicated in haemolytic disease of the newborn. The presence of the G antigen

---

Box 6.4 Apparent inconsistencies in blood grouping and antibody identification due to the presence of the G antigen

In her first pregnancy, JF (a 24-year-old female) had been grouped as O Rh D negative rr (dce/dce) with anti-D antibody in her plasma at a level of 0.67 IU ml^{-1}. Fortunately, her baby had not been affected by her low level of antibody. Unfortunately, the blood group of the father had not been checked during this pregnancy. Twelve months later, JF was again pregnant and attended the antenatal booking clinic on 20 August. She was confirmed as O Rh D negative (rr) with an anti-D level of 1.57 IU ml^{-1}. This time a blood sample was obtained from her husband and he tested as O Rh D positive R$_2$r (DcE/dce).

On 29 October, a routine check indicated that JF had now developed anti-C in addition to anti-D (which was now at a level of 1.95 IU ml^{-1}). Again, on 26 November, anti-C+D was confirmed and by now the anti-D level had risen dramatically to 12.9 IU ml^{-1}. Presumably, the anti-C (and the rising level of anti-D) were due to the baby being both C+ and D+. This was disturbing news for the family in two ways: the rising level of antibody indicated a potential risk to the baby and as the husband was grouped as R$_2$r, and therefore C negative, it appeared that he was not the father of the baby.

JF's anti-D level eventually rose to 20.3 IU ml^{-1} and the baby was born by caesarean section, 6 weeks early in January. The baby was grouped as O Rh D positive R$_2$r (*DcE/dce*) with a strongly positive direct antiglobulin test (see Chapter 10). Fortunately, the baby responded well to phototherapy and mother and baby both made full recoveries. In addition, and of most importance, the baby's Rh type was consistent with the husband being the father.

The explanation for the apparent inconsistencies in blood grouping and antibody identification can be explained by the presence of the G antigen. The cell panels used to identify the mother's antibodies had given positive reactions with all C+ and D+ cells, hence the conclusion that the antibody was anti-C+D and the implication that the husband was not the father (as he was C negative). However, all C+ and D+ cells also carry the G antigen. The husband was R$_2$r (*DcE/dce*) and, although he was C negative, he was G positive. The baby was also R$_2$r and had therefore inherited the father's G antigen. The antibody produced by the mother was in fact anti-G+D.

explains the not uncommon observation that some non-transfused pregnant women apparently produce anti-C+D antibody even though the father of their foetus is found to be C negative (see *Box 6.4*). In such cases, the father has been shown to have passed an R_2 chromosome (DcE) to the foetus. The G antigen would also be expressed by this gene arrangement. Thus, the mother has actually been immunized to produce anti-D and anti-G rather than anti-D and anti-C.

Compound antigens

Not unexpectedly, given that the C/c and E/e antigens are produced by the same gene, antibodies have been described which only react with **compound antigens** that are produced by the same gene. For example, the antibody produced in response to the ce compound antigen is anti-ce (it is also known as anti-f). This antibody will only react with cells expressing both c and e antigens derived from the same gene. This means that anti-ce will react with dce (r) or Dce (R_0) red cells but not with DCe/DcE (R_1R_2) cells where the c and e antigens have been produced by different genes. Other examples of compound antigens with corresponding antibodies are cE, CE and Ce.

6.6   QUANTITATIVE DIFFERENCES IN RH ANTIGENS

Antigen dosage

Dosage is the property displayed when antibodies give stronger reactions in laboratory tests with red cells showing homozygous expressions of the corresponding antigen than with heterozygotes. The dosage effect when the D antigen is reacted with anti-D is not very noticeable as there is considerable overlap in the number of Rh D among the various genotypes. *Table 6.5* gives typical examples of D antigen site numbers for various genotypes and clearly indicates the overlapping of D antigen expression among genotypes.

The replacement of several exon segments from the *RHCE* gene with the equivalent segments from the *RHD* gene can destroy the ability to produce C/c and E/e antigens. Such individuals may only express the D antigen so their phenotype is written as D––. These individuals express much more D antigen on their red cells than those who are normal Rh D positive. A stronger dosage effect is seen with anti-E and anti-c than anti-D, and the most marked effect is seen in antibodies to compound Rh antigens.

Influence of other Rh antigens

The expression of low-frequency antigens often affects the expression of other more common antigens. Low-frequency Rh antigens, for example C^w (RH8) and C^x (RH9), will not be discussed here in detail. However, they are

Table 6.5 The distribution of antigens on red cells

Group	No of antigen sites per cell
DCe/dce (R_1r)	D sites: 9900–14600
Dce/dce (R_0r)	D sites: 12000–20000
DcE/dce (R_2r)	D sites: 14000–16600
DCe/dCe (R_1R_1)	D sites: 14500–19300
DCe/DcE R_1R_2	D sites: 23000–31000
DcE/DcE (R_2R_2)	D sites: 15800–33300
D^ucE/dce (R_2^ur)	D sites: 340–470
D^uCe/D^ucE ($R_1^uR_2^u$)	D sites: 540
D––D––	D sites: 110000–202000
cc	c sites: 70000–85000
cC	c sites: 37000–53000
ee	e sites: 18200–24000
eE	e sites: 13400–14500

usually associated with abnormal expression of one or more of the polymorphic Rh antigens.

In addition, students should be aware of two further effects, commonly known as the *cis* and the *trans* effect.

Cis **effect:** this term is used to describe the observation that when the gene for the D antigen is on the **same** chromosome as a gene for the C or E antigens, the expression of C and E antigens may be depressed. Thus, there is usually more E antigen produced on the red cells of r″ (dcE) than R_2 (DcE) type individuals, and more C antigen on the red cells r′ (dCe) than an R_1 (DCe) type individuals.

Trans **or Ceppellini effect:** this describes the depressed expression of the D antigen which is due to the presence of the gene for the C antigen on the **opposite** chromosome. For example, red cells from an individual who is type R_1r (DCe/dce) will express more D than red cells of the R_0r' (Dce/dCe) type. In some cases, the D antigen may be so depressed as to appear as a weak D (D^u).

Weaker forms of Rh antigens

Amino acid substitutions or exon exchanges to produce *RHD/RHCE* hybrid genes can give rise to gene products and conformational changes which result in altered or weakened expression of common antigens. In addition, some individuals express fewer antigens than normal for no apparent reason. Weak expression of the D antigen arises from the expression of a reduced number of D antigen sites on red cells. The D antigen expressed is the same as that expressed by a normal D-positive person but there is less of it (see *Table 6.5*). This weakened form of D, historically designated D^U, is capable of stimulating the production of anti-D in Rh D-negative individuals. Failure to detect the weakened D antigen in determining the Rh group of blood samples in the transfusion laboratory may result in mis-typing blood donors or neonates as Rh D negative. This could result in an Rh D-negative patient receiving a transfusion of Rh D-positive (D^U) blood or the failure to give anti-D prophylaxis to an Rh D-negative mother with an Rh D-positive (D^U) infant.

6.7   LABORATORY ASPECTS OF RH BLOOD GROUP TYPING

Rh D typing

When undertaking Rh D typing of patients, and when selecting blood donors, consideration must be given to the qualitative and quantitative variations in the expression of the Rh D antigen.

During D typing of patients, it is important to detect all but the very weakest forms in order that the patient is not unnecessarily transfused with Rh D-negative blood, which would be wasteful of a scarce resource. Also, when D typing babies of Rh D-negative women, it is important that the women receive anti-D prophylaxis if the baby has a weak form of D (see also *Box 6.5*).

When D typing donors, it is essential to detect weak forms in order to avoid the chance of transfusing Rh D (weak)-positive donor blood to Rh D-negative patients. This could induce the production of anti-D antibody in the patient.

The detection of partial D types (particularly D^{VI}) is not necessary when typing patients. It is safer to treat them as Rh D negative for transfusion purposes. Patients with a partial D type may produce anti-D antibodies when exposed to normal Rh D-positive donor blood (see Section 6.5).

The partial D expressed on a baby's cells is poorly immunogenic and it is therefore not necessary to offer anti-D prophylaxis to the Rh D-negative mothers of such infants. It is a different approach when D typing blood donors where it is necessary to detect partial D types in order to avoid mistakenly transfusing Rh D (partial)-positive to Rh D-negative patients, as this may result in the induction of anti-D antibody.

Box 6.5   Summary of practical considerations for weak and partial D types

Weak D patients should be treated as Rh D positive.

Partial D patients should be treated as Rh D negative.

Weak D blood donors should be treated as Rh D positive.

Partial D blood donors should be treated as Rh D positive.

Phenotyping and genotyping

It is often necessary to make an assessment of the phenotype and genotype of an individual when selecting blood for transfusion to patients with Rh antibodies, assessing the likely effect on the foetus of a woman's Rh antibodies or when performing family studies. It is usually possible to derive the genotype from information about the phenotype in Rh D-negative individuals. However, it is usually impossible to tell whether Rh D-positive individuals are homozygous or heterozygous for D and therefore their genotype has to be assumed from the statistically most likely arrangement for their ethnic group. The presence of Rh antigens on red cells is most usually detected using the antisera anti-D, anti-C, anti-E, anti-c and anti-e. The phenotype of an individual may be established from the reactions of their red cells when added to these reagents.

Table 6.6 shows an example of the results obtained using Rh antisera and an unknown sample of red cells. Using the example shown in the table, the observed phenotype is DCce. The first assumption is that, as no E antigen was detected, then e antigen must be present on both chromosomes. The second assumption is that, as both C and c antigens were detected, they must be located on opposite chromosomes. Thus, the blood sample is phenotypically **? C e / ? c e**, where **?** = **D** or **non-D (d)** and / divides the two chromosomes.

Table 6.6 Example of the possible genotype of a blood sample using (Caucasian) population frequency statistics

Antisera						Genotype		
-D	**-C**	**-E**	**-c**	**-e**	**Phenotype**	**Most likely**	**Less likely**	**Least likely**
+	+	−	+	+	DCce	*DCe/dce*	*DCe/Dce*	*Dce/dCe*
						R_1r	R_1R_0	R_0r'

+ indicates a positive reaction, − indicates a negative reaction.

The gene for D is either present on both chromosomes, making the phenotype **D C e / D c e** (R_1R_0 = 2% in Caucasians), or on only one chromosome. In the latter case the second chromosome may either carry the gene for C, resulting in the arrangement **D C e / d c e** (i.e. type R_1r, found in 33% of Caucasians) or that for c, giving **D c e / d C e** (i.e. type R_0r', which has a frequency of <1% in Caucasians).

The most likely genotype is *DCe/dce* (R_1r), heterozygous with respect to D, although this is not necessarily the correct one. However, it is important to note that if these results were obtained from an individual of the black population, then the genotype *DCe/Dce* (R_1R_0), homozygous with respect to D, would be the most probable (see *Box 6.6*).

Box 6.6   *Dce* distribution

The gene arrangement *Dce* (R_0) is much more prevalent in black populations than any other population. In fact, it occurs with a frequency of 44% compared with 2% in Caucasian, oriental and Native American populations.

Nature of Rh antibodies

Rh antibodies are usually immune in nature although naturally occurring forms of anti-D, anti-C, anti-E and anti-C^w have been reported. The antibodies may be found in the IgM or IgG form. Anti-D production has even been reported following transfusion of fresh frozen plasma, presumably containing small amounts of red cell membrane. This is due to the highly immunogenic nature of the D antigen (see *Box 6.7*). Antibodies with specificities within the Rh system are often found in cases of autoimmune haemolytic anaemia, e.g. anti-e, anti-C+e, anti-c, anti-c+E (see Chapter 8).

Box 6.7   Immunogenicity of Rh D antigen

The Rh D antigen is the most immunogenic of all the protein antigens. It has been reported that as many as 80% of Rh D-negative individuals receiving a transfusion of Rh D-positive red cells will produce anti-D antibody. Also, up to 16% of Rh D-negative mothers exposed to a foeto-maternal haemorrhage from an Rh D-positive foetus will produce anti-D antibody. Despite the success of anti-D prophylaxis, anti-D is still the most common cause of clinically significant haemolytic disease of the newborn.

Anti-D is the most common of all immune blood group antibodies in Rh D-negative individuals. It is sometimes found in association with anti-C (anti-C+D) or anti-E (anti-D+E), and rarely with both (anti-C+D+E).

In Rh D-positive patients, anti-E is often found in R_1r (*DCe/dce*) and R_1R_1 (*DCe/DCe*) genotypes. Anti-c and anti-c+E are quite common in R_1R_1 patients. Anti-C and anti-e are much less common.

Antibodies to compound Rh antigens (anti-ce, anti-Ce, etc.) may be present in sera containing other Rh antibodies but are difficult to differentiate by routine laboratory tests. Rarely, they may be the sole Rh antibody present in a serum.

Laboratory detection

Immune Rh antibodies often have a wide thermal range. The majority react optimally at 37°C and are best detected using the indirect antiglobulin test or enzyme-treated red cells (see Chapter 10). The naturally occurring forms usually react optimally at lower temperatures. Rh antibodies are not considered to be complement-fixing antibodies but exert their effects by opsonization and antibody-dependent cellular cytotoxicity (ADCC) (see Chapters 2 and 8).

Clinical significance

Rh antibodies may cause immediate or delayed haemolytic transfusion reactions. In addition, anti-D is still the most common cause of severe haemolytic disease of the newborn despite anti-D prophylaxis programmes. Anti-c is also recognized as the cause of a significant number of severe cases of haemolytic disease of the newborn. Rh antibodies are found in many cases of autoimmune haemolytic anaemia. Their deleterious effects cause these antibodies to be of importance in the clinical environment, i.e. they are clinically significant. Antibodies in the Rh system are the most clinically significant of all blood group antibodies apart from the ABO system. The Rh antigens D and c, in particular, are highly immunogenic.

SUGGESTED FURTHER READING

Avent, N.D. and Reid, M.E. (2000). The Rh blood group system: a review. *Blood* **95**, 375–387.

Avent, N.D., Madgett, T.E., Lee, Z.E., Head, D.J., Maddocks, D.G. and Skinner, L.H. (2006) Molecular biology of Rh proteins and relevance to molecular medicine. *Expert Reviews in Molecular Medicine* **8**, 1–20.

BCSH Blood Transfusion Task Force (2004) Guidelines for compatibility procedures in blood transfusion laboratories. *Transfusion Medicine* **14**, 59–73.

Carritt, B., Kemp, T.J and Poulter, M. (1997) Evolution of the human RH (rhesus) blood group genes: a 50 year old prediction (partially) fulfilled. *Human Molecular Genetics* **6**, 843–850.

Jones, J., Scott, M.M. and Voak, D. (1995) Monoclonal anti-D specificity and Rh D structure: criteria for selection of monoclonal anti-D reagents for routine typing of patients and donors. *Transfusion Medicine* **5**, 171–184.

Sonneborn, H.H and Voak, D. (1997) A review of 50 years of the Rh blood group system. *Biotest Bulletin* **5**, 389–552.

Telen, M.J. (1996) Erythrocyte blood group antigens: polymorphisms of functionally important molecules. *Seminars in Hematology* **33**, 302–314.

Van Kim, C., Colin, Y. and Cartron, J. (2006) Rh proteins: key structural and functional components of the red cell membrane. *Blood Reviews* **20**, 93–110.

Wagner, F.F., Gassner, C., Muller, T.H., Schonitzer, D., Schunter, F. and Flegel, W.A. (1999) Molecular basis of weak D phenotypes. *Blood* **93**, 385–393.

Westhoff, C.M. (2007) The structure and function of the Rh antigen complex. *Seminars in Hematology* **44**, 42–50.

SELF-ASSESSMENT QUESTIONS

1. Describe the *cis* and *trans* effects in relation to the expression of Rh antigens.
2. Name the genes and their products for the 'two-locus model' for the Rh genes.
3. List the five major antigens of the Rh system.
4. What is the thermal range and mode of detection for immune Rh antibodies?
5. Why is it not necessary to detect partial D types when performing routine Rh blood grouping on patients?
6. If a patient has *RHD* and *RHCe* genes on one chromosome and *RHD* and *RHcE* genes on the opposite chromosome, how would you write the patient's genotype using the Fisher notation?

Other blood group systems

Learning objectives
After studying this chapter you should be able to:
■ List the cellular functions of the blood group antigens
■ Outline the general features of the Lewis, P, Ii, MNS, Lutheran, Kell, Kidd and Duffy blood group systems
■ Describe the clinical and laboratory significance of the blood group antibodies in transfusion, pregnancy and haemolytic disease of the newborn
■ List the antigen frequencies in the white and black population for the selected blood groups

The blood group systems covered in this chapter will be the carbohydrate-based systems Lewis, P and Ii, and the protein-based systems Kidd, Kell, Duffy, Lutheran and MNS. At the level of this introductory text, only certain key features (see *Box 7.1*) for each of these other blood group systems will be described.

Box 7.1 Key features to be considered for other blood group systems

Antigens
Their frequency; general features such as whether they are present on red cells at birth; any dosage effect or variability of expression; and any disease associations.

Antibodies
Whether they are immune or naturally occurring; which immunoglobulin class they belong to and their frequency; the preferred method of detection; their ability to bind complement; and their clinical significance in relation to transfusion reactions or haemolytic disease of the newborn.

7.1 CARBOHYDRATE ANTIGENS

Lewis system (ISBT 007, symbol LE)

The antigens Le^a and Le^b are not the products of a pair of allelic genes as the nomenclature might suggest. Indeed, they are not true red cell antigens. Lewis antigens are synthesized in secretory tissue, such as gut epithelium, and released into the plasma as soluble glycolipids. They are adsorbed onto the red cell surface from the plasma. The ability to secrete soluble Lewis antigen is independent of the ability to secrete ABH soluble antigens (see also *Box 7.2*). ABH secretion is controlled by a separate secretor (*Se* or *FUT2*) gene (see Chapter 5). The Lewis gene (*Le* or *FUT3*), which is located on chromosome 19, codes for the production of a transferase enzyme (fucosyl transferase), which attaches fucose to the subterminal position of type 1 precursor oligosaccharide. This monofucosylated structure is the Le^a antigen.

In secretory tissue, when the *Se* (*FUT2*) gene is present, the *H* (*FUT1*) gene produces a transferase which attaches fucose to the terminal position of type 1 precursor oligosaccharide. This is soluble H antigen. The Lewis transferase then acts by adding a further fucose at the subterminal position of the soluble H antigen. This difucosylated structure is the Le^b antigen.

Box 7.2 Interactions between ABH and Lewis transferases in secretory tissue

In secretory tissue, the soluble A and B antigen structures may act as substrates for the Lewis transferase, producing the compound antigens ALe^b and BLe^b.

A, B and Lewis transferases all compete for the soluble H antigen structure, so that there is usually less Le^b substance produced, and therefore less expressed on red cells in group A, B and AB individuals than in group O individuals.

When the *Se* (*FUT2*), *H* (*FUT1*) and *Le* (*FUT3*) genes are present, the type 1 precursor has fucose added at the terminal position by H transferase, and at the subterminal position by Lewis transferase, to produce Le^b antigen (see *Fig. 7.1*). In the absence of the *Se* (*FUT2*) gene, the Lewis transferase adds fucose to the subterminal position to produce Le^a antigen. Thus, all Le(b+) individuals are ABH secretors and all Le(a+) individuals are ABH non-secretors.

Individuals who lack any Lewis antigen may be considered as homozygous for point mutations in the *Le* (*FUT3*) gene, which produces inactive

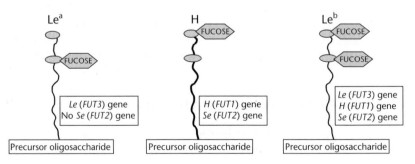

Figure 7.1
Structures of H and Lewis antigens.

Table 7.1 Summary of interactions between *Se (FUT2), Le (FUT3)* and *H (FUT1)* genes

Genotype	Antigens in plasma			Lewis phenotype on red cells
	ABH	**Leᵃ**	**Leᵇ**	
SeSe or *Sese* *LeLe* or *Lele* *HH* or *Hh*	+	+ small amount	+	Le(a–b+)ˉ
Sese *LeLe* or *Lele* *HH* or *Hh*	–	+	–	Le(a+)
SeSe or *Sese* *LeLe* or *Lele* *Hh*	–	+	–	Le(a+)
Sese *LeLe* or *Lele* *Hh*	–	+	–	Le(a+)
SeSe or *Sese* *lele* *Hh* or *Hh*	+	–	–	Le(a–b–)
sese *lele* *HH* or *Hh*	–	–	–	Le(a–b–)
SeSe or *Sese* *lele* *hh*	–	–	–	Le(a–b–) ,
Sese *lele* *hh*	–	–	–	Le(a–b–)

transferase. Their genotype is usually designated *lele*. Whether they secrete soluble ABH antigen will depend on whether or not they carry a *Se (FUT2)* gene (see *Table 7.1*). As described above, Lewis antigens are soluble antigens secreted into plasma and reversibly adsorbed onto red cells. This means that Lewis antigen can be lost from red cells when blood samples are stored. When testing cells for Lewis antigen or sera for Lewis antibodies, it is therefore advisable to use the freshest available red cells. Similarly, because the Lewis antigen is found in plasma and the supernatant suspending medium of stored red cells, cells must be washed in saline prior to testing to avoid the soluble antigen neutralizing Lewis antibody in the test or typing serum.

Lewis system antigens

The Lewis antigens are produced in secretory tissue. They also appear as soluble antigens in plasma and are reversibly adsorbed onto red cells. The Lewis antigens may weaken or disappear during pregnancy and this is thought to be due to the change in the lipoprotein composition of blood. Sometimes Lewis antibodies are also detected in the plasma. However, these antibodies disappear when the normal Lewis phenotype is restored after the birth of the infant.

The **Le^a** antigen, discovered in 1946, shows variable expression from individual to individual and is unstable on storage. Le^a antigen is not detected on newborn red cells, but 80–90% of infants appear Le(a+) as they mature from a few weeks to 6 months. They begin to express their true Lewis type with increasing age. The Le^a substance may be taken up from plasma onto Le(a–) red cells making them appear Le (a+).

The **Le^b** antigen, discovered in 1948, is weak or absent at birth and is not readily detected on red cells until 3 years of age; also it is unstable on storage. The Le^b substance may be taken up from plasma onto Le(b–) cells.

Table 7.2 Population frequency of Lewis system antigens

	Frequency in population (%)	
	White	**Black**
Le(a+b–)	22	23
Le(a–b+)	72	55
Le(a–b–)	6	22

Table 7.3 Clinical and laboratory features of Lewis system antibodies

	Anti-Le^a	**Anti-Le^b**
Immune or naturally occurring	Naturally occurring in Le(a–b–) individuals	Naturally occurring in Le(a–b–) and rarely in Le(a+b–) individuals
Immunoglobulin type	Usually IgM	IgM
Frequency	Common antibody	Common antibody
Detection	Readily detected with enzyme tests Usually a cold agglutinin, but may be a 37°C agglutinin	Readily detected with enzyme tests Usually a cold agglutinin, but may be a 37°C agglutinin
Complement binding	May bind complement May cause *in vitro* haemolysis of Le(a+) cells	Some examples bind complement
Haemolytic transfusion reaction (HTR)	May cause HTR	Unlikely to cause HTR
Haemolytic disease of the newborn (HDN)	Does not cause HDN	Does not cause HDN
General	Usually of low titre Classically show stringy agglutination of red cells	Usually of low titre Classically show stringy agglutination of red cells

Le^b antigens are more easily detected on red cells from blood groups O and A_2 than from blood group B, although they are more difficult to detect on red cells from blood groups A_1 and A_1B. This is due to competition from A and B transferases for the H antigen. *Table 7.2* indicates the frequency of Lewis antigens in the population, while *Table 7.3* illustrates the features of Lewis antibodies.

Presence of the Le^b antigen is associated with the development of peptic ulcers and stomach cancer. This is thought to be due to the fact that the Le^b antigen, expressed on the cells of the mucosal surface of the stomach, acts as a receptor for *Helicobacter pylori*. This microorganism has been isolated from the stomach of some patients who suffer from gastritis and appears to cause peptic ulcers and cancer.

P system (ISBT 003, symbol P1) and globoside collection (ISBT 209, symbol GLOB)

Discovered in 1927 by Landsteiner and Levine during animal experiments, the P antigen system has proved to be more complex than the Lewis system.

As with all the carbohydrate antigens, the sugars which express the different antigens of the P system are attached to a precursor oligosaccharide by the action of glycosyl transferase enzymes. At the time of writing, the molecular basis underlying these transferases is unknown. The antigens to consider are P_1, P and P^k.

P_1 is now considered to be the only true antigen of the P system, the antigens P and P^k having been assigned to the globoside collection by the ISBT. The P^k antigen is produced by the action of a transferase which adds galactose to a ceramide dihexose (CDH) precursor, converting it to a ceramide trihexose (CTH). The P antigen is produced by the action of a transferase which adds *N*-acetyl galactosamine to CTH, converting it to a globoside (see *Fig. 7.2*). The addition of these P sugars makes the P^k antigen

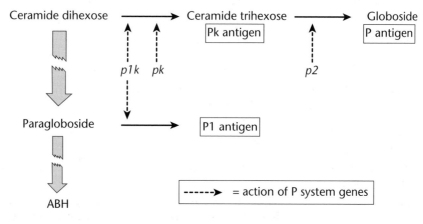

Figure 7.2
Development of P system antigens.

less accessible to its antibody, which may explain why P^k is difficult to detect on P+ red cells in the laboratory. The P_1 antigen is produced by the action of a transferase that adds galactose to a paragloboside precursor. This precursor is closely related to both CDH and the precursor oligosaccharide chain of the ABH antigens. *Fig. 7.2* shows the development of the P system antigens. The P system genes and their products are described in *Table 7.4*, while *Table 7.5* shows the P system antibodies.

Table 7.4 Genes and gene products of the P system, based on Graham and Williams two-locus model

Gene	Allele	Gene product	Action
Locus 1	p^k	α-Galactosyl transferase	Converts CDH to CTH (P^k)
	p^{1k}	α-Galactosyl transferase	Converts CDH to CTH (P^k)
			Converts paragloboside to P_1
	p	None	None
Locus 2	p^2	β-Galactosyl transferase	Converts CTH (P^k) to globoside (P)
	p^{20}	None	None

Table 7.5 Clinical and laboratory features of P system antibodies

	Anti-P$_1$	Anti-P	Anti-PP$_1$P^k (Tj^a)
Immune or naturally occurring	Naturally occurring	Naturally occurring	Naturally occurring
Immunoglobulin type	IgM	IgM	IgM
Frequency	Common in P$_1$ individuals	Found in rare P^{k+} individuals	Found in rare pp individuals
Detection	Cold agglutinin Readily detected using enzyme tests	Wide thermal range Readily detected using enzyme tests	Wide thermal range Readily detected using enzyme tests
Complement binding	A few examples bind complement at 37°C	Most bind complement at 37°C Some are haemolytic	Most bind complement at 37°C and cause haemolysis at 37°C
Haemolytic transfusion reaction (HTR)	May cause HTR if complement bound at 37°C	May cause HTR if complement bound at 37°C	May cause HTR
Haemolytic disease of the newborn (HDN)	Does not cause HDN	Does not cause HDN	Does not cause HDN
General	**Auto-anti-P** may be found as the biphasic IgG associated with paroxysmal cold haemoglobinuria. It binds to red cells in the cold and causes haemolysis when warmed to 37°C		

Table 7.6 P system phenotypes, antigens and antibodies

Phenotype	Antigens	Possible antibodies	Frequency in population (%)
P_1	P_1 and P	–	White 79, black 93
P_2	P	Anti-P_1	White 21, black 7
p	–	Anti-PP_1P^k	Rare
P_1^k	P_1 and P^k	Anti-P	Very rare
P_2^k	P^k	Anti-P, anti-P_1	Rarest

P system antigens

The frequency of the P_1 antigen in white populations is 79% and in black populations is 93% (see *Table 7.6*). The P_1 antigen shows variable expression on red cells from weak to very strong in different individuals. The P_1 antigen is not fully expressed on foetal and neonatal red cells. Both P_1 and P^k substance have been found in the fluid derived from the hydatid cyst, which develops following infection with the migratory tapeworm *Echinococcus granulosus*. P_1 substance has been found in red cells, plasma, droppings from pigeons and in the white of turtle doves' eggs.

P system antigens have been found on urinary tract epithelium where they may act as receptors for microorganisms such as *Escherichia coli* and so play a role in the pathogenesis of some cases of urinary tract infection and pyelonephritis. In addition, the P antigen is the cellular receptor for parvovirus B19, a virus which causes erythema infectiosum in children. It may be transmitted in blood and, in rare cases of haemolytic anaemia, may inhibit red cell production.

Ii system (ISBT 207, symbol I)

Discovered in 1956 by Wiener and associates, I and i have common related structures. They are both high-frequency antigens whose expressions are inversely proportional. Foetal and neonatal red cells express the i antigen with little detectable I antigen. During the first 18 months of life, the expression of i slowly decreases and that of I increases.

The I and i antigens are defined by a series of carbohydrates on the inner portion of ABH oligosaccharide type 2 precursor chains. I is expressed by the branched structure and i by the linear structure. The i antigen is synthesized by the action of β-3-*N*-acetylglucosaminyl transferase and β-4-*N*-acetylgalactosyl transferase on the paragloboside-derived precursor chain (see *Fig. 7.2*). The i antigen is converted to the I structure by the branching enzyme β-6-*N*-acetylglucosaminyl transferase. As branched chains form, anti-i no longer has good access to its antigen and therefore i antigen expression appears to decrease as I antigen develops.

Most adult red cells express large amounts of I antigen and very little i antigen. Rarely, adult red cells continue to express i antigen rather than I antigen. This may be due to the inability to produce the branching enzyme due to a recessive trait. Two types of adult i phenotype have been described: i_1, which has the least amount of i antigen expression, is associated with white populations, whilst i_2, which has a little more i antigen expression, is associated with black populations.

The I and i antigens are widely distributed throughout the body, having been found on lymphocytes, granulocytes, monocytes and platelets, as well as on red cells. The antigens have also been found in saliva, milk, plasma, amniotic fluid, urine and ovarian cyst fluid. Thus, normal adults are positive for the I antigen (I+) and neonates are positive for the i antigen (i+).

The clinical and laboratory features of the antibodies in the Ii system are shown in *Table 7.7*. For further discussion of the role of Ii antibodies in autoimmune haemolytic disease, see Chapter 8.

Compound carbohydrate antigens

The biochemical structures that define ABH, Lewis, P and Ii antigens are very similar. It is therefore not surprising that many antibodies have been described which react with compound antigens from these carbohydrate antigen systems. Examples of these compound antigens are ALe^b, BLe^b, IA, IB, IH, iH, IP_1, iP_1 and ILe^{bH}. The antibodies to these compound antigens require both antigens to be present for the antibody to react.

7.2   PROTEIN ANTIGENS

Due to lack of space and the introductory nature of this book, only the most common, clinically significant or historically important antigens will be considered for each blood group system below.

MNS system (ISBT 002, symbol MNS)

There are 43 antigens in this system, four of which, M, N, S and s, will be considered in this section. The antigens M and N were discovered in 1927 during experiments in which human red cells were injected into rabbits to elicit an immune response. The S antigen was discovered in 1947 and the s antigen in 1951. These antigens were detected in human blood using the indirect antiglobulin technique (IAT). The antigens M, N, S and s are produced by two, co-dominant allelic pairs of genes, *GYPA* and *GYPB*, occurring at two closely linked loci on chromosome 4. The gene combinations which encode the antigens MS, Ms, NS and Ns are inherited intact, due to the close linkage of the gene loci, and can be traced through families. The antigen combination MS is more common than Ms and Ns is more common than NS. The M and N antigens are expressed on red cell

Table 7.7 Clinical and laboratory features of the antibodies in the Ii system

	Auto-anti-I	Auto-anti-i
Immune or naturally occurring	Naturally occurring	May be found secondary to infections such as infectious mononucleosis, or diseases involving the reticulo-endothelial system
Immunoglobulin type	IgM	IgM (rarely IgG)
Frequency	Present in all normal sera	See above
Detection	Enhanced in enzyme tests Cold agglutinin May be ABO group specific Identified by titration against adult and cord red cells. Anti-I will react with both adult and cord red cells, but to a much higher titre with adult red cells	Enhanced in enzyme tests Cold agglutinin Identified by titration against adult and cord red cells. Anti-i will react with both adult and cord red cells, but to a much higher titre with cord red cells
Complement binding	May bind complement and cause haemolysis *in vitro*	May bind complement
Haemolytic transfusion reaction (HTR)	May cause HTR	
Haemolytic disease of the newborn (HDN)	Does not cause HDN	May cause mild HDN
General	Most common auto-antibody found in cold haemagglutinin disease. May be very high titre with extended thermal range May be found with raised titre secondary to infection, especially *Mycoplasma pneumoniae* **Allo-anti-I:** naturally occurring cold agglutinin in the very rare adult I-negative individuals	

glycophorin A (GPA) and the S and s antigens on glycophorin B (GPB). The antigens differ due to a different amino acid sequence on the N-terminal portion of GPA and GPB. The glycophorins are sialoglycoproteins, which contribute greatly to the net negative charge of the red cell membrane. This negative charge prevents red cells from adhering to one another or to vessel walls. It seems possible that GPA acts as an assembly point for the biosynthesis of red cell membrane proteins such as Band 3 protein and that GPB plays a similar role in the assembly of the Rh complex.

The MNSs antigens are well developed on the red cells at birth. They show a marked dosage effect when present in the homozygous state. The antigens of the MNS system are destroyed by treatment with enzymes in the laboratory (see Chapter 10).

Table 7.8 Population frequency of the MNSs antigens

	Frequency in population (%)	
	White	**Black**
M+N–	28	26
M+N+	50	44
M–N+	22	30
M–N–	Rare	Rare
S+s–	11	3
S+s+	44	28
S–s+	45	69
S–s–	0	<1

The population frequency of the MNS system antigens is shown in *Table 7.8*. The clinical and laboratory features of the MNS system antibodies are summarized in *Tables 7.9 and 7.10*.

Glycophorin A (MN glycoprotein) acts as a receptor for the malarial parasite *Plasmodium falciparum* and red cells lacking GPA have long been noted to resist invasion by this organism.

Lutheran system (ISBT 005, symbol LU)

There are 20 antigens in or associated with the Lutheran system. Only two, Lu^a discovered in 1946 and Lu^b discovered in 1956, will be described in this

Table 7.9 Clinical and laboratory features of MN system antibodies

	Anti-M	**Anti-N**
Immune or naturally occurring	Naturally occurring	Naturally occurring
Immunoglobulin type	IgM and IgG	IgM and IgG
Frequency	Fairly common	Very rare
Detection	Usually cold agglutinin May act in IAT at 37°C Not detectable with enzymes Reactions often enhanced at pH below 6.5	Usually cold agglutinin May act in IAT at 37°C Not detectable with enzymes
Complement binding	Unlikely to bind complement	Unlikely to bind complement
Haemolytic transfusion reaction (HTR)	May cause HTR if reactive at 37°C	May cause HTR if reactive at 37°C
Haemolytic disease of the newborn (HDN)	May cause mild HDN	May cause HDN

Table 7.10 Clinical and laboratory features of Ss system antibodies

	Anti-S	Anti-s
Immune or naturally occurring	Immune	Immune
Immunoglobulin type	IgG and IgM	IgG
Frequency	Uncommon antibody	Uncommon antibody
Detection	May act as a cold agglutinin Best detected in IAT at 37°C Variable reactions with enzymes	Best detected in IAT at 37°C Variable reactions with enzymes
Complement binding	May bind complement	May bind complement
Haemolytic transfusion reaction (HTR)	May cause HTR	May cause HTR
Haemolytic disease of the newborn (HDN)	May cause mild to severe HDN	May cause mild to severe HDN

text. The Lutheran antigens are expressed on red cell membrane glycoprotein structures, which probably play a role in cell adhesion during erythropoiesis. The co-dominant allelic genes *Lu^a* and *Lu^b* are closely linked to the *FUT2 (Se)* gene locus on chromosome 19. This linkage was the first example of autosomal gene linkage in humans to be described. The minus/minus phenotype, Lu(a–b–), in which neither Lu^a nor Lu^b antigen is expressed on the red cell, may arise by one of three mechanisms, namely, by the inheritance of an unlinked, dominant inhibitor gene *In(Lu)*, by the inheritance of a silent (*lu*) gene from both parents, or by the inheritance of a recessive, sex-linked inhibitor gene, *XS2*.

The Lutheran system antigens show variable expression among individuals. They are poorly developed at birth and poorly immunogenic. The population frequency for the Lutheran system is shown in *Table 7.11*. The clinical and laboratory features of antibodies to the Lutheran system are summarized in *Table 7.12*.

In sickle cell disease, the Lu glycoprotein may mediate the adhesion of sickle cells to the vascular endothelium. This adhesion appears to be regulated by the phosphorylation of Lu glycoprotein by protein kinase A.

Table 7.11 The population frequency of the Lutheran system antigens

	Frequency in population (%)	
	White	Black
Lu(a+b–)	0.15	0.1
Lu(a+b+)	7.5	5.2
Lu(a–b+)	92.35	94.7
Lu(a–b–)	Rare	Rare

Table 7.12 Clinical and laboratory features of Lutheran system antibodies

	Anti-Lu^a	Anti-Lu^b
Immune or naturally occurring	Naturally occurring or immune	Immune
Immunoglobulin type	IgM and IgG	IgM and IgG
Frequency	Not very common	Rare
Detection	May act as cold agglutinins May act in IAT at 37°C Variable reactions with enzymes	May act as cold agglutinins Most act in IAT at 37°C Variable reactions with enzymes
Complement binding	May bind complement	May bind complement
Haemolytic transfusion reaction (HTR)	Unlikely to cause HTR	May cause HTR
Haemolytic disease of the newborn (HDN)	May cause mild HDN	May cause mild HDN
General	Mixed field agglutination	Mixed field agglutination

Kell system (ISBT 006, symbol KEL)

The Kell system antigens are expressed on a red cell membrane glycoprotein with membrane-bound enzyme activity (zinc endopeptidase). There are 22 antigens in or associated with the Kell system of which six will be considered. They are the co-dominant, allelic pairs K and k, Kp^a and Kp^b, and Js^a and Js^b. These three pairs of alleles are closely linked on chromosome 7.

The antigen K, originally called Kell, was discovered in 1946. It was named after Mrs Kellacher who developed an antibody in her plasma which reacted with the red cells of her husband, her elder daughter and her newborn infant. In 1949, k, also known as Cellano, was discovered, followed by Kp^a, also known as Penney, in 1957. Two further antigens in the system, Kp^b, also known as Rautenberg, and Js^a, also known as Sutter, were discovered in 1958. The antigen Js^b, also known as Matthews, was discovered in 1963. Kp^a is associated with Caucasian and Js^a with black populations.

Individuals who express both K and Kp^a antigens always carry the corresponding *K* and *Kp^a* genes on different chromosomes. The presence of the Kp^a antigen has been shown to suppress the expression of k and Js^b antigens.

There is a rare, silent, recessive gene, K_0, which produces no Kell antigens. Individuals who are of $K_0 K_0$ genotype express no Kell antigens and if immunized by exposure to a Kell antigen, may produce an antibody known as anti-K$_U$. It is not certain whether this antibody reacts with a 'total' or 'universal' Kell antigen, or is a mixture of many Kell antibodies. The presence of the K_0 gene on one chromosome depresses the expression of Kp^a by the opposite chromosome (*trans* effect). There is also a sex-linked gene, *XK*, which encodes the antigen K$_X$. Although K$_X$ is not a Kell system antigen, its presence is required for the normal expression of Kell antigens. XK and Kell proteins are linked, close to the membrane surface, by a single disulphide bond. Although primarily expressed in erythroid tissues, Kell and XK are also present in many other tissues.

K is the most immunogenic antigen outside the ABO and Rh systems. Kell system antigens are well developed at birth and Kell system antigens show some dosage effect but this is not very marked or consistent.

Table 7.13 shows the population frequency of the antigens in the Kell system. The clinical and laboratory features of the antibodies are summarized in *Table 7.14*.

The McLeod phenotype has both weakened Kell as well as K_x antigens and occurs in males. The red cell phenotype is only one aspect of the **McLeod syndrome**, which includes a variety of muscular and neurological defects, elevated serum creatine phosphokinase and acanthocytic red blood cells (cells with thorny projections, see *Fig. 7.3*).

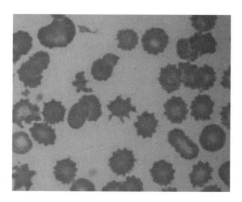

Figure 7.3
Acanthocytes in peripheral blood.

Table 7.13 The population frequency of the Kell system antigens

	Frequency in population (%)	
	White	**Black**
K+k–	0.2	<0.1
K+k+	8.8	3.5
K–k+	81	96.5
Kp(a+b–)	<0.1	<0.1
Kp(a+b+)	2	<0.1
Kp(a–b+)	98	>99
Js(a+b–)	0.1	1
Js(a+b+)	0.1	18
Js(a–b+)	>99	81

Table 7.14 Clinical and laboratory features of Kell system antibodies

	Anti-K	Anti-k (Cellano)
Immune or naturally occurring	Immune	Immune
Immunoglobulin type	IgM and IgG	IgM and IgG
Frequency	Common in transfused patients	Rare
Detection	Variable results in enzymes May act as a cold agglutinin Usually best detected in IAT at 37°C	Variable results in enzyme Best detected in IAT at 37°C
Complement binding	May bind complement	May bind complement
Haemolytic transfusion reaction (HTR)	Causes HTR	Causes HTR
Haemolytic disease of the newborn (HDN)	Causes HDN	Causes HDN

	Anti-Kpª (Penney)	Anti-Kpᵇ (Rautenberg)
Immune or naturally occurring	Immune	Immune
Immunoglobulin type	IgG	IgG
Frequency	Rare	Very rare
Detection	Variable results in enzyme tests Best detected in IAT at 37°C	Variable results in enzyme tests Best detected in IAT at 37°C
Complement binding	May bind complement	May bind complement
Haemolytic transfusion reaction (HTR)	Causes HTR	Causes HTR
Haemolytic disease of the newborn (HDN)	Causes HDN	Causes HDN

	Anti-Jsª (Sutter)	Anti-Jsᵇ (Matthews)
Immune or naturally occurring	Immune	Immune
Immunoglobulin type	IgG	IgG
Frequency	Rare	Very rare
Detection	Variable results in enzyme tests Best detected in IAT at 37°C	Variable results in enzyme tests Best detected in IAT at 37°C
Complement binding	May bind complement	May bind complement
Haemolytic transfusion reaction (HTR)	Causes HTR	Causes HTR
Haemolytic disease of the newborn (HDN)	Causes HDN	Causes HDN

Chronic granulomatous disease (CGD) is a rare X-linked or autosomal recessive disorder of the superoxide-generating enzyme NADPH oxidase. Phagocytic cells are not able to respond with respiratory burst during phagocytosis and so do not generate superoxide, which impairs their ability to kill catalase-positive microorganisms such as staphylococci (see Chapter 1).

The X-linked condition (60% of cases) is caused by mutations or deletions of the *CYBB* gene. Large deletions in the region of the X-linked *CYBB* gene are known to delete adjacent genes, such as *XK*, the gene that controls the expression of the Kell blood group antigen. Patients with CGD who have this gene deletion can become sensitized to Kell antigens after red blood cell transfusion. For this reason, the Kell antigen status in CGD patients requiring blood transfusion should be examined carefully.

Duffy system (ISBT 008, symbol FY)

The Duffy blood group antigens are expressed on a red cell membrane glycoprotein with chemokine receptor activity. The Fy glycoprotein is also known as Duffy Antigen Receptor for Chemokines (DARC). The Duffy gene (*DARC*) is located on chromosome 1. Of the six antigens in the Duffy system, only the co-dominant, allelic pair Fy^a and Fy^b will be considered. The Fy^a antigen was discovered in 1950 and Fy^b in 1951. The minus/minus phenotype, Fy(a–b–), which lacks the Fy protein, occurs in individuals homozygous for the silent gene *Fy*. This phenotype is very rare in white populations but occurs in 68% of black populations of African descent and results from a point mutation in the Duffy gene. The Duffy antigens are interesting in that they are the site of attachment to the red cell for the malarial parasites *Plasmodium vivax* and *P. knowlesi*. Thus, possession of the Fy(a-b-) genotype is advantageous to those living in areas where malaria is endemic.

The population frequency of the Duffy system antigens is shown in *Table 7.15*. The antigens are well developed at birth and are moderately immunogenic. The Fy glycoprotein is expressed on red cells, the endothelial cells of capillary and post-capillary venules, the epithelial cells of kidney collecting ducts, in lung alveoli and in the Purkinje cells of the cerebellum. The clinical and laboratory features of antibodies in the Duffy system are summarized in *Table 7.16*. It should be noted that, in laboratory tests, the antigens are destroyed using enzyme techniques (see Chapter 10).

Table 7.15 The population frequency of the Duffy system antigens

	Frequency in population (%)	
	White	Black
Fy(a+b–)	17	9
Fy(a+b+)	49	1
Fy(a–b+)	34	22
Fy(a–b–)	0	68

Table 7.16 The clinical and laboratory features of the Duffy system antibodies

Features	Anti-Fy^a	Anti-Fy^b
Immune or naturally occurring	Immune	Immune
Immunoglobulin type	IgG	IgG
Frequency	Not uncommon in transfused patients	Rare
Detection	Not detectable using enzyme techniques Best detected in IAT at 37°C	Not detectable using enzyme techniques Best detected in IAT at 37°C
Complement binding	May bind complement	May bind complement
Haemolytic transfusion reaction (HTR)	May cause HTR	May cause HTR
Haemolytic disease of the newborn (HDN)	May cause HDN	May cause HDN

Kidd system (ISBT 009, symbol JK)

The Kidd blood group antigens are expressed on a red cell transmembrane glycoprotein which transports urea across the red cell membrane. The Kidd gene (*SLC14A1*) is located on chromosome 18. There are three antigens in the Kidd system, of which only the co-dominant, allelic genes encoding the Jk^a and Jk^b antigens will be described here. The Jk^a antigen was discovered in 1951 and Jk^b in 1953.

The minus/minus phenotype, Jk(a–b–), occurs in individuals who are homozygous for the silent gene *Jk* or carry the dominant inhibitor gene *In(Jk)*. The silent gene can result from splice-site or missense mutations or partial gene deletions. This phenotype is rare in both black and white populations (see *Table 7.17*).

In laboratory red cell agglutination tests, a marked dosage effect can be demonstrated between homozygous and heterozygous individuals. The Kidd antigens are well developed in the newborn and can be detected on their red cells. The antibodies of the Kidd system are described in *Table 7.18*.

Table 7.17 The population frequency of the Kidd system antigens

	Frequency in population (%)	
	White	**Black**
Jk(a+b–)	27	57
Jk(a+b+)	50	34
Jk(a–b+)	23	9
Jk(a–b–)	Rare	Rare

Table 7.18 The clinical and laboratory features of the Kidd system antibodies

	Anti-Jk^a	Anti-Jk^b
Immune or naturally occurring	Immune	Immune
Immunoglobulin type	IgM and IgG	IgM and IgG
Frequency	Not uncommon in transfused patients	Less common than anti-Jk^a
Detection	Enhanced in enzyme tests Best detected in IAT at 37°C	Enhanced in enzyme tests Best detected in IAT at 37°C
Complement binding	Bind complement	Bind complement
Haemolytic transfusion reaction (HTR)	May cause HTR Common antibody in cases of delayed HTR	May cause HTR
Haemolytic disease of the newborn (HDN)	May cause mild HDN	May cause mild HDN
General	Unstable on storage of blood samples Antibody levels in patients often fall very quickly	Unstable on storage of blood samples Antibody levels in patients often fall very quickly

7.3 IMPORTANCE OF OTHER BLOOD GROUPS IN TRANSFUSION SCIENCE

It is necessary for the transfusion scientist to be aware of the importance of the blood groups described in this chapter. The detection of antibodies in transfused patients who have been given ABO- and Rh-compatible blood products is usually due to the transfusion of red cells containing antigens from one of the above blood group systems. Tests must then be performed to identify the antibodies and knowledge of the antibody characteristics is required. An awareness of the clinical significance of the antibody is important in issuing compatible blood for transfusion in order to prevent unwanted reactions (see Chapter 11). Consideration of the frequency of the antigen in the population is also necessary, for example in selecting suitable blood for transfusion which lacks a particular antigen. There are many important aspects for discussion relating to blood group systems. This chapter has examined some of them at an introductory level.

SUGGESTED FURTHER READING

Avent, N.D. (1996) Human erythrocyte antigen expression: its molecular bases. *British Journal of Biomedical Science* **54**, 16–37.
BCSH Blood Transfusion Task Force (2004) Guidelines for compatibility procedures in blood transfusion laboratories. *Transfusion Medicine* **14**, 59–73.

Daniels, G. (2002) *Human Blood Groups*. Oxford: Blackwell Publishing.

Daniels, G., Poole, J., de Silva, M., Callaghan, T., MacLennan, S. and Smith, N. (2002) The clinical significance of blood group antibodies. *Transfusion Medicine* **12**, 287–295.

Moulds, J.M., Nowicki, S., Moulds, J.J. and Nowicki, B.J. (1996) Human blood groups: incidental receptors for viruses and bacteria. *Transfusion* **36**, 362–374.

Reid, M.E. and Lomas-Francis, C. (2004) *The Blood Group Antigen Facts Book*, 2nd edn. San Diego: Academic Press.

Serum, Cell and Rare Fluid Exchange:
http://balder.prohosting.com/scarfex/index.html

Telen, M.J. (1996) Erythrocyte blood group antigens: Polymorphisms of functionally important molecules. *Seminars in Hematology* **33**, 302–314.

The Bristol Institute For Transfusion Sciences and The International Blood Group Reference Laboratory: http://www.blood.co.uk/ibgrl

SELF-ASSESSMENT QUESTIONS

1. Which antigens are carbohydrate structures?
2. Which antigens are proteins structures?
3. Describe how the I and i antigens differ.
4. List the antibodies which are able to bind complement to red cells.
5. Which blood groups have a connection with malaria?

Immune and autoimmune haematology disorders

Learning objectives

After studying this chapter you should be able to:

■ Describe the effects of antibody attachment on red blood cells

■ Define immune and autoimmune haemolytic anaemia

■ Define three mechanisms of immune haemolytic anaemia due to drugs

■ Describe the underlying mechanisms of the disorders

■ Describe the role of the maternal response in haemolytic disease of the newborn

■ Describe how haemolytic disease of the newborn affects the foetus or neonate

■ Outline the methods used to establish the presence of immune disorders

■ Outline the strategies for prophylaxis of haemolytic disease of the newborn

■ Describe autoimmune thrombocytopenic purpura

8.1 MECHANISMS OF RED CELL DESTRUCTION

A brief explanation of the mechanisms of red cell destruction is needed to understand the significance of inappropriate red cell antibody production and the clinical consequences to patients. Normal red cell breakdown occurs in the liver and spleen (extravascular) when the cells become aged or damaged. The haemoglobin is further degraded into its components haem and globin. The molecules of haem are converted to bilirubin, which is degraded by the liver. Thus, the possibility of free haemoglobin or its products in the circulating blood is avoided. When red cell breakdown occurs inside the blood vessels, i.e. intravascularly, mechanisms exist for the removal of free haem by binding to haptoglobin. This is to prevent subsequent damage to the kidneys. Haptoglobins are proteins which are found in normal plasma. As they bind to haem, the levels of free circulating haptoglobins are reduced. The haem–haptoglobin complex is removed from the circulation by the reticuloendothelial (RE) system. Raised blood levels of breakdown products, such as bilirubin, haem or haemoglobin itself suggest haemolysis of red cells due to a pathological defect. These may be estimated by the laboratory to investigate a possible haemolytic episode. A raised bilirubin level is evident in a patient as the yellow skin colour of jaundice. Immune and autoimmune red cell antibodies may attach to the corresponding antigenic component on the red cell membrane, sometimes involving the fixation of complement components as well (see Chapter 3). This results in inappropriate red cell breakdown, which may be intravascular or extravascular.

Box 8.1 Mechanisms of intravascular and extravascular haemolysis

Intravascular
Complement-mediated haemolysis
Via classical pathway
• Recognition unit C1q, C1r, C1s
• Activation unit C4, C2, C3
• Membrane attack unit C5, C6, C7, C8, C9
The clinical consequences are free circulating haemoglobin, which leads to renal failure and disseminated intravascular coagulation.

Extravascular
Macrophage-mediated red cell destruction
• Phagocytosis and/or antibody-dependent cellular cytotoxicity
• Sub-haemolytic complement fixation
• Splenic sequestration of red cells
• Macrophage receptors for IgG, Fc and complement
The result is a release of damaged and C3d-coated red cells.

As red cell destruction is increased, the bone marrow responds by increasing the release of immature red cells into the circulation. This is demonstrated in the peripheral blood film by the presence of nucleated red cells, reticulocytes and/or polychromasia, all of which indicate the presence of immature red cells. When the bone marrow no longer has the capacity to compensate, anaemia develops in the patient, as shown by a lowered red cell count and haemoglobin level. In circumstances when the increase in haemolysis is extravascular, it is detectable by increased plasma bilirubin levels and the presence of free haemoglobin in the patient's plasma (haemoglobinaemia). In addition, there may be haemoglobin in the urine (haemoglobinuria) in severe cases. The haemolysis in immune/autoimmune haemolytic anaemia is said to be 'extrinsic', meaning that the defect causing the premature destruction of the red cells is extrinsic to the red cell. This type is therefore differentiated from the 'intrinsic' causes of haemolytic anaemia, such as thalassaemia or sickle cell disease, in which the defect is an abnormality of the red cell.

8.2 CAUSES AND CLASSIFICATION OF IMMUNE HAEMOLYTIC ANAEMIA

Immune haemolytic anaemia (IHA) may occur as a result of production of an antibody in response to a foreign stimulus, for example, a blood transfusion which is incompatible, or drug treatment. Autoimmune haemolytic anaemia (AIHA) is caused by an abnormal process taking place in the patient's own body, resulting in the production of autoantibodies. Antibody production may be stimulated by disease processes, the presence of malignant cells or substances produced during a disease. The disorders are called **primary** or **idiopathic** if no apparent cause for their existence can be identified and **secondary** if the cause is known. Those IHAs which are drug induced have a special category and will be described in more detail later. Autoimmune haemolytic anaemia is classified into two types according to the temperature at which the antibodies react optimally with red cells. This is called the **thermal range**. In the **warm-type** of AIHA, an antibody is produced that combines with the red cells at any temperature but most rapidly at 37°C. *Colour plate 2* shows haemagglutination in peripheral blood caused by autoantibodies present in a patient with IHA.

Cold-type AIHA antibodies combine optimally at 0–20°C and show a decreased affinity to attach to the red cells as the temperature increases.

The most useful test for the laboratory detection of antibodies bound to red cells *in vivo* is the direct antiglobulin test (DAT), also called the Coombs test, which is described in Chapter 10. The DAT must be positive to confirm the presence of antibodies on the red cell membrane.

8.3 HAEMOLYTIC TRANSFUSION REACTIONS

A haemolytic transfusion reaction is one of the major hazards of blood transfusion and will also be discussed in Chapter 11; however, the mechanism will be briefly outlined here. This type of reaction occurs in a patient who has been transfused with blood which contains antigens foreign to the patient's own red cells, or antigens to which the patient has previously produced antibodies. These latter are either from a previous transfusion or from pregnancy during which a haemorrhage of foetal red cells into the maternal circulation has occurred.

Haemolytic reactions that take place during or within 24 hours of transfusion are described as 'acute', whereas those occurring a few days later are 'delayed'. As haemolysis takes place, it may be either intravascular or extravascular. Usually, acute haemolytic reactions are intravascular and delayed reactions are extravascular. The mechanism is as follows: first, the antibodies produced will bind to antigens on the transfused red cells. Secondly, if the antibodies are 'complement fixing', then complement proteins will also be bound or 'fixed' to the red cell membrane. Thirdly, this activation of complement leads to membrane damage and the damaged red cells are recognized by phagocytes, engulfed and removed from the circulation. An example of ABO incompatibility is one of the most severe incidents.

Blood group O recipients of transfused blood which is from blood group A or B donors possess antibodies to A and B, usually of immunoglobulin types IgG and IgM, and possess the ability to bind complement. In addition, the antigens A or B on transfused red cells are very immunogenic, and thus will induce a strong antibody response in the recipient. This situation results in rapid haemolysis with serious, often fatal, consequences for the patient.

8.4   WARM AUTOIMMUNE HAEMOLYTIC ANAEMIA

Warm AIHA occurs as a result of a patient producing antibodies against their own red cells. These antibodies react with red cells most optimally at 37°C. The pathophysiology is that red cells are coated with an antibody, usually IgG type, which may also have the ability to bind complement to the red cells. Thus, the red cells are phagocytosed by macrophages and removed from the circulation. As the red cells become more damaged, they lose part of the membrane and lose their shape, becoming spherical. Such cells are recognized in a peripheral blood smear as spherocytes. Cell destruction occurs in the spleen or liver, i.e. organs of the RE system.

The incidence of warm AIHA varies. Primary cases, that is, those which are not due to the existence of another disorder, account for 48% of all cases, whereas drug-induced IHA is relatively rare at approximately 8%. Diseases causing secondary AIHA include lymphomas, systemic lupus erythematosus (SLE), rheumatoid arthritis, pernicious anaemia, hepatitis and colitis, as well as miscellaneous causes. The incidence in females is greater than in males. Some of the known disease associations for warm and cold types will be further described.

Warm antibody types

AIHA in children. This is usually an acute disease following viral infection. Most patients recover, but a few develop a condition which persists, usually associated with deficiencies of immunoglobulin such as IgA.

AIHA with thrombocytopenia. In such cases, an IgG-type antibody develops which is specific for platelet antigens.

AIHA and tumours. Tumours of the ovaries and thymus may cause AIHA, although this is rare. The relationship between the tumour and auto-antibody production is unclear. However, removal of the tumour seems to cure the disorder.

AIHA secondary to diseases. SLE sufferers may develop a red cell auto-antibody and 10% show a positive DAT. The antibody type is IgG, is complement fixing, and occasionally shows Rh specificity. Hodgkin's disease and lymphoma patients may produce an auto-antibody which is also capable of fixing complement to the red cells; thus, a few cases are DAT positive. Similarly, a small number of patients with chronic lymphocytic leukaemia (CLL) are DAT positive as they have produced an IgG antibody that is probably of the Rh type.

Box 8.2 Rare intravascular haemolysis caused by IgA auto-antibodies

A 66-year-old man was admitted to hospital and investigated for muscle cramps in his legs, extreme breathlessness, and severe weight loss. For 2 weeks prior to admission, he had noticed that his urine was brown. On clinical examination, he appeared pale and jaundiced. His blood pressure, pulse rate and temperature were normal. The laboratory tests demonstrated severe intravascular haemolysis. His haemoglobin level was very low, the plasma bilirubin level was raised at 103 μmol l^{-1} and hapto-globins were low at less than 0.6 g l^{-1}. Examination of a peripheral blood smear showed raised retic-ulocytes, erythroblasts and spherocytes. However, laboratory results included a negative direct antiglobulin test (Coombs test) using a standard reagent containing anti-IgG and the complement components anti-C3c and anti-C3d. This was initially confusing for the diagnosis. However, his red cells were then tested using a monospecific anti-IgA antiglobulin reagent and this time found to be strongly positive. The next step was to elute (i.e. 'wash off ') antibodies from his red cells and test these auto-antibodies to see if they were IgA type. The results of the eluate confirmed the presence of an IgA antibody, which was found to be specific for the Rh antibody anti-e. The patient was diagnosed as a case of warm AIHA and treated with blood transfusions using blood which was type e negative. The case is unusual in that the DAT, testing for IgG-type antibodies and complement components on the red cells, was negative. Antibodies were only demonstrated when tested for the presence of IgA-type. Warm AIHA caused by antibodies of immunoglobulin class A (IgA) are very rare. The patient responded to treatment with blood transfusions to correct his anaemia and prednisone to subdue his immune response, and gradually his symptoms disappeared.

8.5 COLD HAEMOLYTIC ANAEMIA

Chronic cold haemagglutinin disease accounts for approximately 45% of cold antibody-type immune disorders. Infectious mononucleosis (glandular fever) is caused by the Epstein–Barr virus and accounts for about 30% of cases, while other disorders such as lymphoma and paroxysmal cold haemo-globinuria are also implicated. These will be described below.

Chronic cold haemagglutinin disease

The antibody which is present in these patients is an IgM that is specific for the I antigen found on all adult red cells. IgM always activates complement and is thus very haemolytic. Antibody binding to the patient's red cells occurs when the patient's skin temperature drops below 28–30°C. Haemoglobinuria, haemosiderinuria, haemoglobinaemia and jaundice occur as a result of intravascular haemolysis. However, the haemolysis of red cells only occurs when the peripheral circulation (such as in fingertips and toes) is restored to body temperature as the blood becomes warm. The antibody dissociates from the red cells at 37°C but the activated complement components are still attached. If haemolysis does not occur immediately, then the complement-coated red cells will be removed by the RE system (see Chapters 1 and 3).

Cold auto-antibodies and infection

The presence of cold auto-antibodies may be due to infection, particularly with *Mycoplasma pneumoniae*. This causes an acute haemolytic anaemia due to the anti-I antibody, which has a high thermal range. In infectious mononucleosis, only a few cases develop haemolysis, and this is related to the patient producing **high-titre** anti-i auto-antibodies which react with their red cells at cold temperatures. Adult red cells exhibit the I antigen (see Chapter 7) and are not usually affected by anti-i. The reason why a small number of patients develop haemolysis is not clear.

Paroxysmal cold haemoglobinuria

Paroxysmal cold haemoglobinuria (PCH) is a rare condition in which the thermal range of the antibody is 15–17°C. This means that there must be considerable chilling before haemolysis of the red cells begins. The antibody is known as the Donath–Landsteiner antibody (named after the workers who first described it in 1904) and it activates complement. Acute anaemia develops rapidly as haemoglobin is freed from red cells haemolysing in the blood vessels and is lost in the urine (haemoglobinuria). This is one of the consequences of intravascular haemolysis. A secondary condition may occur, usually associated with viral infection, in which the patient sustains one attack of haemolysis and the antibody titre in their plasma falls within a week. The antibody in PCH appears to be of anti-P specificity and is of the IgG class. It has a biphasic action in that it attaches to red cells at cold temperatures, such as that in cold fingers and toes, but red cell breakdown occurs as complement is fixed to the cell membrane at normal body temperature. It is extremely haemolytic to the patient's red cells.

8.6   UNDERLYING MECHANISMS WHICH MAY CAUSE IMMUNE/AUTOIMMUNE HAEMOLYTIC ANAEMIA

There are a number of possible mechanisms which could contribute to the antibody production in IHA/AIHA patients:

Genetic factors. Although the incidence of familial AIHA is low, some cases do occur and thus it is likely that a genetic predisposition to develop AIHA exists.

Modified red cell antigens. It is possible that viruses, bacteria or some metabolite could enter the red cell membrane or expose hidden antigens, thus giving rise to antibodies reactive with the red cell surface.

Cross-reacting antibodies. These are antibodies associated with infection, which may also cause AIHA. The auto-antibody in these cases is short-lived and is polyclonal, suggesting a response to an infection.

Failure to recognize and eliminate auto-reactive clones. Many different antibody specificities are generated by rearrangements and mutations of the immunoglobulin genes in developing B lymphocytes as they mature. The result is a series of lymphocytes which can form distinct antigen-recognition units on their cell surface and these recognition units can compete for specific antigens. It is thought that auto-reactive lymphocytes, which are capable of proliferating into clones of plasma cells producing auto-antibody, are eliminated or paralysed during the establishment of tolerance.

Auto-antibodies may arise as a result of proliferation of clones of lymphocytes to which tolerance could not be established or maintained.

8.7 DRUG-INDUCED HAEMOLYTIC ANAEMIA

The drug-induced haemolytic anaemias may be divided into two main types. The first type induce the formation of antibodies directed against the drug (or metabolite), or some drug/protein complex. These are known as the immune haemolytic anaemias and the antibody can be detected only if the drug is present. The second type induces the formation of antibodies against antigens on the red cell membrane and the presence of the drug is not required for antibodies to be detected. This type produces a haemolytic anaemia which is caused by an auto-immune antibody. Drugs are low molecular mass substances and are not likely to induce antibodies directly. However, they are transported in the body by a firm chemical coupling of the drug to a protein carrier. The protein which acts as the carrier may or may not be a component of the tissue which is damaged by the resulting anti-drug antibody formed. Four methods are described to explain the mechanisms by which the drugs induce antibody formation.

Immune complex mechanism

This is also called the **innocent bystander mechanism**. Most of the drugs which induce antibodies act by this method. Common examples are quinine, quinidine, *p*-aminosalicylic acid and phenacetin. An antibody is produced which then combines with the drug, and the 'drug–antibody complex' attaches to the cell surface. This induces the binding of complement to the red cells and so haemolysis occurs (see *Fig. 8.1*). Thus, the protein carrier allows the drug to act as a hapten (see Chapter 1). It has been suggested that either the drug is bound to the cell membrane of the

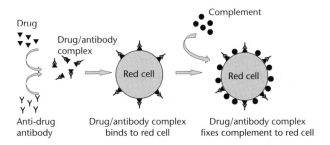

Figure 8.1

The immune complex mechanism. Anti-drug antibodies form a complex with the drug which then bind to the red cell membrane. This causes complement to be bound to the red cell and leads to haemolysis.

target cell, or that a drug/plasma protein complex is formed. It seems that IgM antibodies are associated with the destruction of red cells and IgG antibodies with platelet destruction as far as quinidine is concerned. Platelets have Fcγ receptors but red cells do not. However, red cells have C3b receptors that facilitate the uptake of complement-coated complexes.

Even a small quantity of drug will result in a rapid intravascular haemolysis in a sensitive person. It appears that these immune complexes bind reversibly to the target cells and can migrate from cell to cell, fixing complement at each stop. This would explain the massive effect of small amounts of drug. The antibody is usually IgM, though can be IgG, and binds complement.

Drug adsorption (hapten) mechanism

This mechanism differs in that drugs, such as penicillin and cephalothin, are strongly bound to the red cell membrane and are present on the cells of all patients taking large doses of the drug. This coating is not damaging in itself, but some patients develop high-titre antibodies which attack the cell-bound penicillin and result in haemolysis. The major hapten (see Chapter 2) in penicillin is the benzylpenicilloyl (BPO) group and over 90% of normal patients contain anti-BPO antibodies. In most cases, these antibodies are IgM, but those associated with haemolytic anaemia are IgG. Large doses of penicillin and cephalothin are required for antibodies to be induced, the rate of haemolysis develops more slowly and it is not intravascular. The antibody is usually of the IgG class and complement is not involved. *Fig. 8.2* illustrates the basis of the drug adsorption mechanism.

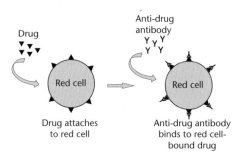

Figure 8.2
The drug adsorption mechanism. The drug attaches directly to the red cell membrane by adsorption. Antibodies to the drug are produced and bind to the red cell-bound drug.

Drug-induced haemolytic anaemia caused by methyldopa

AIHA associated with methyldopa occurs in approximately 20% of patients treated for raised blood pressure with the drug methyldopa (Aldomet). Patients develop a positive DAT due to the formation of an IgG antibody.

A small number develop haemolytic anaemia. The DAT may continue to be positive up to 18 months after stopping the drug treatment. The antibody shows Rh specificity, usually anti-c or anti-e.

Membrane modification or non-immunological protein adsorption

This mechanism involves the non-specific adsorption of plasma proteins onto the membrane of red cells which have been sensitized by the drug, for example cephalothin. These proteins include IgG, IgM, IgA, the acute phase proteins α_1-antitrypsin, α_2-macroglobulin, fibrinogen and complement components C3 and C4. This adsorption may not lead to haemolytic anaemia, but it can confuse the results when a patient is investigated, as the DAT becomes positive. The mechanism is shown in *Fig. 8.3*.

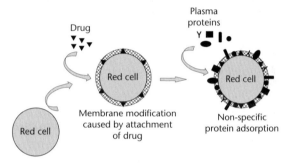

Figure 8.3
The membrane modification mechanism. Attachment of the drug to the red cell membrane modifies it in such a way that non-specific plasma proteins are also adsorbed.

Cephalothin is unique among drugs in that it can cause a positive DAT by three different mechanisms. As well as the mechanism previously described, anti-cephalothin antibodies may be produced as described for penicillin, or cephalothin-coated red cells may cross-react with anti-penicillin antibodies.

8.8 LABORATORY TESTS FOR DIAGNOSIS OF AUTOIMMUNE/IMMUNE HAEMOLYTIC ANAEMIA

In order to diagnose AIHA, it is necessary to show in the laboratory that:

- the antibody present in the patient's serum sample has been bound *in vivo* to the patient's red cells. This would be shown by a positive DAT. In addition, after eluting the antibody, i.e. removing it from the red cells, it has a specificity which makes it capable of agglutinating red cells of other individuals with the same phenotype

- the patient's red cells have a shortened life span; this indicates that active haemolysis is occurring
- the antibodies are present in the patient's serum and are similar to those on the patient's red cells

Sometimes not all of these criteria may be met, for example cold antibodies may only be detectable by their ability to activate complement. Alternatively, the auto-antibody may not show any specificity or it may be reacting with a drug. Finally, a positive DAT may be found without anaemia if the patient has been able to compensate for the haemolysis by a response in the bone marrow to increase red cell production.

8.9 HAEMOLYTIC DISEASE OF THE NEWBORN

Many years ago, it was not uncommon for an infant to be stillborn. One of the common causes for the failure of these infants to survive was described in 1939 by Philip Levine and Rufus Stetson (see *Box 8.3*). They described the passage of antibodies from the mother to the foetus and the syndrome was later defined as 'Rh haemolytic disease of the newborn'.

Box 8.3 The first report of haemolytic disease of the newborn

Philip Levine and Rufus Stetson published a paper in the *Journal of the American Medical Association* called 'An unusual case of intra-group agglutination', the findings of which were not considered to be particularly significant at that time. However, the paper was reprinted some 40 years later in *Vox Sanguinis* (1980) and hailed as a milestone in the history of medical science.

Prior to treatment, 1 in 200 pregnant mothers developed Rh antibodies and a fifth of these lost their infants in the first pregnancy, the rate increasing dramatically in subsequent pregnancies to just over half of the infants surviving. Haemolytic disease of the newborn (HDN) (and of the foetus) is caused by production of an antibody in the mother in response to an antigen carried on the red blood cells of the developing baby. If some trauma occurs during the pregnancy and the baby's red cells cross into the mother's circulation, it is known as a **transplacental haemorrhage (TPH)** or a **foetomaternal haemorrhage (FMH)**. This can also occur as a normal consequence of birth. The placental barrier excludes antibodies of the IgM class but will allow IgG antibodies to cross due to the presence of Fc receptors on the cell membrane of the placental cells to which the antibodies bind. The antibody produced by the mother is actively transported across the placenta into the foetal circulation by these receptors. The antibody then attaches to the foetal red cells and causes haemolysis to occur in the foetal circulation. This can result in HDN, depending upon a number of factors. The strength of the antibody which is developing in the maternal circulation must be regularly checked so that steps can be taken to prevent or

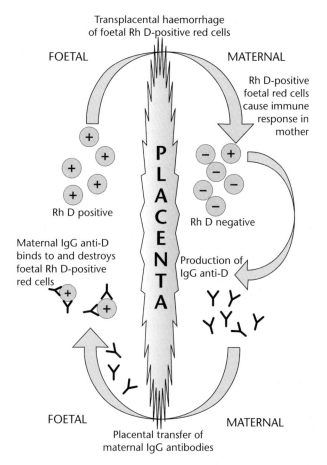

Figure 8.4
Haemolytic disease of the newborn in a Rh D-positive foetus and Rh D-negative mother. Foetal red cells which are RhD positive enter the maternal circulation. Anti-D is produced by an immune response in the Rh D-negative mother. The IgG anti-D crosses the placenta into the foetal circulation and attaches to the foetal red cells causing haemolysis.

minimize the effects of the antibody in the foetal blood. An illustration of how HDN occurs is shown in *Fig. 8.4*. An antibody is described as high titre when the serum containing the antibody is diluted in the laboratory, usually by a series of doubling dilutions in saline, and shows agglutination at dilutions greater than 1 in 32 with red cells expressing the corresponding antigen.

Clinical effects of haemolysis on the foetus or neonate

The attachment of IgG antibodies to the foetal red cells results in their sensitization and destruction by the RE system. The foetus or neonate suffers from the events that occur during intravascular haemolysis. The haemoglobin levels fall due to decreased red cell survival and serum bilirubin levels are raised.

These are regularly measured by the laboratory. Bilirubin is a breakdown product of haemoglobin so this is an indication of how much haemolysis is taking place in the baby's circulation. If the levels of unconjugated bilirubin become too high, the result will be brain damage due to **kernicterus** (see *Box 8.4*). In this situation, the baby may be placed under a source of ultraviolet light to speed up the breakdown of bilirubin. Normal adult levels of unconjugated bilirubin are less than 18 μmol l^{-1} although in normal newborn infants the level may reach 85 μmol l^{-1}. Levels of 350 μmol l^{-1} or more are not uncommon and are highly toxic to the brain. The levels of bilirubin are more of a problem after the baby is born because prenatally it is cleared via the placenta. The neonatal liver is not sufficiently mature to conjugate the bilirubin and render it non-toxic. In this instance, it may be necessary to exchange the total blood volume of the baby with fresh donor blood. An exchange transfusion has a number of beneficial effects and is straightforward to perform.

If the baby is severely affected prior to birth, the result is intrauterine death from **hydrops foetalis**. Hydrops foetalis is a condition which causes stillbirth. The foetus is very pale and swollen with fluid in the body cavity and brain, which results in mental damage and death. In its moderate form, the disease results in the baby being born with severe anaemia and jaundice. Mildly affected babies show a slight anaemia and possibly some jaundice.

Box 8.4 Kernicterus

Kernicterus comes from the words kernel and icterus. Kernel, meaning nucleus in German, refers to brain and icterus (Latin) refers to the yellow pigment, in this case due to bilirubin. Bilirubin has an affinity for the lipids present in the brain tissue and therefore causes damage, particularly in babies.

Test to detect antibodies formed by the mother

Although HDN can be caused by a number of IgG antibodies, the most frequently described antibody involved in HDN is the Rh antibody, anti-D. It is an IgG antibody and is therefore likely to cause foetal damage if produced. Mothers who are Rh D negative lack the D antigen on their red cells. However, if the father is Rh D positive, the D antigen may be inherited by the baby. A father who is homozygous for the *RHD* gene can only pass the gene for the D antigen to the baby, which will then be heterozygous for the *RHD* gene and, thus, for the production of the D antigen. However, if the father is Rh D positive and heterozygous for the *RHD* gene, the baby is equally likely to inherit the D-positive genotype as the D-negative genotype. Thus, it is useful to identify the genotype of the father to see if there is a likelihood that the baby is carrying the *RHD* gene. The mother is then checked regularly throughout her pregnancy for the production and level of antibodies. If the titre of antibodies rises to a dangerous level in her circulation, then clearly the foetus is at risk (see *Box 8.5* for a guide to risk levels). As a rough guide, anti-D levels greater than 4 IU ml^{-1} are indicative of risk. However, it is important to note that a number of factors are involved such as the mother's previous obstetric history, how fast the development of antibodies has occurred and the type or

---

Box 8.5 Clinically significant levels for anti-D and anti-c

Levels of anti-D detected in maternal blood
<4 IU ml^{-1}: HDN is unlikely
4–15 IU ml^{-1}: moderate risk of HDN
>15 IU ml^{-1}: high risk of hydrops foetalis

Levels of anti-c detected in maternal blood
<7.5 IU ml^{-1}: continue to monitor levels
7.5–20 IU ml^{-1}: risk of moderate HDN; refer to specialist unit
>20 IU ml^{-1}: risk of severe HDN; refer to specialist unit
It is important to note that anti-c may cause delayed anaemia in the neonate.

---

subclass of IgG involved. Tests on the foetus include **amniocentesis** to withdraw some amniotic fluid from the foetal sac through a needle inserted into the abdominal wall of the mother. The bilirubin pigment may be measured in the fluid using a spectrophotometer. This gives an estimation of the amount of red cell destruction taking place. The Rh (D) status of the foetus can be identified using the technique of **chorionic villus sampling** during the first 3 months of pregnancy to obtain a sample of foetal cells. Chorionic villus sampling involves taking a sample from the placenta and can be performed from the 8th week of pregnancy. Alternatively, the Rh (D) status can be detected using cell-free foetal DNA, which is present in a blood sample taken from the mother, and testing for the presence of the *RHD* gene by **polymerase chain reaction methods**. Other techniques for assessing the foetus are foetal blood sampling using cordiocentesis, and amniocentesis to estimate levels of antibodies in the amniotic fluid. Maternal and foetal red cells may be tested using techniques such as **flow cytometry** and **chemiluminescence** (see *Box 8.6*). Once antibodies have been detected, it is important to monitor the foetus using **velocimetry**, a measurement of the speed of blood flow through the middle cerebral artery of the foetus. The technique used to do this is **Doppler ultrasonography**. If the velocity of blood flow is increased, it indicates anaemia in the foetus.

Box 8.6 Antibody levels during pregnancy

Haemolytic disease of the newborn is most often associated with the development of anti-D. Anti-C, unlike anti-D, is an antibody not often found in pregnancy. It has been reported that anti-C was present in only 2% of referred antenatal patients. Anti-D (or anti-C+D) was found in 20% and anti-c in 12%. When anti-C does occur, it usually has little, if any, clinical effect. Guidelines for antenatal testing currently recommend the identification and titration of clinically significant red cell antibodies at the time the expectant mother first books into the antenatal clinic and again at 28 weeks of pregnancy. If the antibody titre is found to be greater than 1 in 32, there is deemed a greater risk of HDN in the foetus. However, the correlation between titre and disease severity is generally poor. The chemiluminescence test (CLT) has been shown to give better correlation of outcome for Rh antibodies than the titre of antibodies. A CLT index of greater than 20% is indicative of haemolytic disease in the foetus, although this test cannot be totally relied on as a predictor of HDN.

Exchange transfusion

As stated earlier, it may be necessary to replace the baby's blood with fresh blood. This may be performed as a prenatal or postnatal procedure. The donor blood selected for exchange transfusion must be less than 5 days old and have a haematocrit of approximately 0.8 to 0.9 (see Chapter 9). The blood should be irradiated to inactivate the donor lymphocytes in order to minimize the risk of transfusion-related graft-versus-host disease in the foetus or neonate. Blood for transfusion is checked for compatibility by cross-matching with the maternal serum. The technique is performed by removing small volumes of the neonatal or foetal blood and simultaneously infusing donor blood. The beneficial effects of exchange transfusion are as follows: circulating antibodies and sensitized red cells are diluted or removed, the haemoglobin level is raised to a normal level and the bilirubin levels are lowered, thus preventing further risk of damage. The British Committee for Standards in Haematology has produced guidelines for the transfusion of neonates. See *Box 8.7* for a case study description of abnormal antibody production and intrauterine transfusion.

Box 8.7 HDN caused by anti-C

A 32-year-old pregnant woman booked into the antenatal clinic and her blood group was performed. She was typed as OR_2r (DcE/dce). The prenatal antibody screen was performed and the titre of anti-C was measured at 1 in 64. The antibody level remained the same at 28 weeks of pregnancy, increasing to 1 in 128 at 4 weeks post-intrauterine death of the foetus. Despite this, the CLT index at this time was only 3% and tests were performed to exclude the presence of an antibody to a low-frequency antigen carried on the foetal red cells. The conclusion for this case was that hydrops foetalis had occurred due to an unusual anti-C. After two further miscarriages, the patient eventually had a successful pregnancy, although the infant did require an exchange transfusion. In view of this patient's history and because the CLT appeared unreliable in detecting anti-C, serological methods together with physical monitoring of the foetal health were carried out. The foetus was monitored using middle cerebral artery (MCA) Doppler ultrasound, and an early delivery was planned. During this last pregnancy, the use of the MCA Doppler was invaluable as it indicated the need for repeated interuterine transfusions, with the result of a live birth. This is a rare case of anti-C causing severe HDN and illustrates the importance of testing for antibody production during pregnancy. It also demonstrates the poor predictive value of antibody titration in pregnancy and the use of alternative techniques.

Prophylactic disease prevention

Prophylaxis, i.e. prevention, stops a disease occurring before the events which cause it have happened. The prophylaxis of HDN has been a great success story (see *Box 8.8*).

Rh prophylaxis with anti-D has dramatically reduced the number of deaths due to HDN and the number of registered deaths for this disorder in England and Wales fell from 106 in 1977 to 11 in 1990. It is recommended

---

Box 8.8 Prophylaxis of HDN

Professor Sir Cyril Clarke was famous for his work at Liverpool University during the 1960s on the mechanics of Rh sensitisation in red blood cells. His workers had noted a correlation between the incidence of sensitisation by Rh antibodies in maternal blood samples and the number of foetal red cells in the mother's circulation. The Rh negative mothers became sensitised by small amount of foreign (foetal) Rh positive blood during their pregnancy. It has also been noted that Rh sensitisation was much reduced when there was incompatibility of the ABO group between mother and baby, for example, a group O mother and group A father, resulting in a group A baby. It was reasoned that the naturally occurring anti-A (or anti-B) destroyed the foetal cells as soon as they entered the mother's circulation. Thus, the mother was less likely to become sensitised to Rh D positive cells. Therefore, to introduce anti-D into the mother's blood would have the same effect as the anti-A or anti-B, that is, to destroy Rh D positive cells. In a clinical trial, the expected result was found, i.e. that the mother did not become sensitised and her immune system was not be stimulated to produce anti-D. A group of American workers published similar findings using a passive anti-D to prevent active immunisation on exposure to the antigen. They found too that this procedure had a protective effect.

---

that a standard dose of 500 IU (100 mg) immunoglobulin is routinely given to all Rh D-negative mothers at 28 weeks and 34 weeks of pregnancy. This is sufficient to destroy the red cells resulting from a foetal maternal haemorrhage (FMH) of less than 4 ml of foetal blood. Larger doses are required if the FMH has been greater. The way in which the volume of foetal blood is estimated is described later. In order to be effective, it is important that prophylactic anti-D is given to mothers of all Rh-positive babies within 72 hours of giving birth and to all Rh-negative pregnant women following amniocentesis, chorionic villus sampling, miscarriage, induced abortion, ectopic pregnancy or any trauma to the abdomen. Each of these events is likely to cause FMH. The mechanism of action of prophylactic anti-D is that it attaches to the foetal Rh D-positive circulating cells in the mother, which are then trapped in the spleen.

Quantitation of foetal maternal haemorrhage

There is a variety of methods to determine whether FMH has occurred and to estimate the amount of foetal red cells in maternal blood.

A standard formula used to determine the volume of FMH is based on the number of foetal cells multiplied by the maternal blood volume and divided by the number of maternal cells. In order to estimate the number of foetal cells, the most popular test is still the Kleihauer–Betke stain, which was first described in 1957. This is a simple technique based on the principle that the haemoglobin in foetal cells (HbF) is resistant to elution out of the red cells when placed in an acid environment. In contrast, the haemoglobin contained in adult red cells (HbA) is removed by the action of an acid pH. In the Kleihauer–Betke stain, a smear of maternal blood is placed in a solution of haematoxylin and hydrochloric acid to lower the pH to about 1.5, and then counterstained with eosin. The result is that the mater-

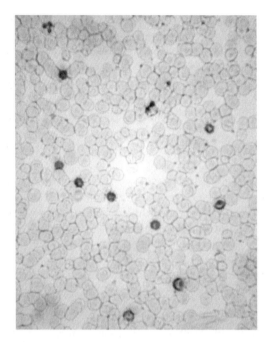

Figure 8.5
Kleihauer–Betke stain of maternal blood depicting foetal cells stained dark and
maternal cells as 'ghost' cells.

nal red cells appear as 'ghost' cells, with only the red cell stroma remaining,
but foetal cells stain a deep pink and leucocytes stain blue/grey. The ratio
of foetal to maternal red cells is counted under a microscope and the extent
of foetal haemorrhage can be calculated (see *Fig. 8.5*). Other methods for
determining the number of foetal cells include flow cytometry and
immunofluorescence (see Chapter 13). These techniques are usually more
time-consuming and expensive but highly accurate. The technique of flow
cytometry is based on the detection and quantification of fluorescent
markers attached to red cells containing HbF. As HbF is bound to Rh D-
positive cells, it is presumed to be foetal in origin, although this is not necessarily the case. For example, maternal blood from thalassaemia patients or
those with hereditary persistence of HbF (a rare syndrome) would confuse
the results. Another limitation of this method is that it cannot detect Rh D-
negative foetal cells.

Some automated haematology analysers are able to measure immunofluorescence and may be increasingly incorporated as a tool for the measurement of FMH in hospital laboratories.

Other antibodies and haemolytic disease of the newborn

The most common incompatibility is ABO incompatibility between mother
and foetus but it does not cause problems *in utero* and usually only causes
mild anaemia post-delivery. If the mother produces IgG anti-A or anti-B in

response to the baby's A, B or AB red cells, then these antibodies are able to cross the placenta and damage the foetal cells in the same way. ABO incompatibility can occur in the first pregnancy and any further pregnancies. Haemolysis can also occur due to the action of other IgG antibodies and occasionally anti-C, anti-c, anti-E, anti-e, anti-K or anti-Fy^a may be implicated as well as various other irregular antibodies. There are approximately four deaths per year in the UK from HDN caused by anti-c or anti-K. The pathogenesis of HDN due to anti-K is a slightly different mechanism in that the anaemia is caused by suppressed red cell production rather than haemolysis.

The success of anti-D immunoprophylactic treatment has meant that there are more occurrences of mild or moderate HDN due to non-Rh D antibodies. Sometimes the symptoms do not develop in these infants until a few days after birth so it is important to screen for antibodies in pregnant women who may be at risk.

8.10 IMMUNE DISORDERS AFFECTING PLATELETS

Autoimmune thrombocytopenic purpura

The immune mechanism for the disorder in which platelets are destroyed by antibodies is similar to that of red cells as previously described. Autoimmune thrombocytopenic purpura (AITP) is characterized by the production of auto-antibodies against platelets. This results in the individual having a reduced number of circulating platelets. As platelets have an important function in the prevention of haemorrhage, a lack of platelets results in the development of **purpura**, which are visible on the skin and similar to bruising. Acute AITP usually occurs in children after an infection. Chronic AITP is more commonly seen in adults, although both are very rare disorders.

Alloimmune thrombocytopenic purpura

Neonatal alloimmune thrombocytopenic purpura (NAITP) is also rare and this disorder is seen in newborn infants born with pupuric rash and a tendency to bruising and bleeding. The pathological mechanism is similar to that of HDN, in that in this situation antibodies are produced by the mother against the platelet antigens of the foetus. As a result, foetal platelets are destroyed by the phagocytes of the RE system. Alloimmune thrombocytopenia can also occur as a result of platelet transfusions. The process is similar to an incompatible transfusion due to red cell antigens and antibodies, but in this case is due to a mismatch of platelet antigens between donor and patient. *Box 8.9* shows some common platelet antigens and the corresponding type of platelet membrane glycoprotein. You are encouraged to read a haematology textbook for further details about platelet membrane structure and platelet antigens.

Box 8.9 Common human platelet antigen (HPA) types		
System	Antigen	Glycoprotein (GP)
HPA-1	HPA-1a HPA-1b	GPIIIa
HPA-2	HPA-2a HPA-2b	GPIbα
HPA-3	HPA-3a HPA-3b	GPIIb
HPA-4	HPA-4a HPA-4b	GPIIIa
HPA-5	HPA-5a HPA-5b	GPIa
HPA-15	HPA-15a HPA-15b	CD 109

Mechanism of platelet antibody destruction

The role of T cells has been implicated in identifying the cause of antibody production. Clones of T cells have been found in AITP patients. Autoreactive T and B cells are stimulated to produce auto-antibodies, which then opsonize platelets. Phagocytosis is enhanced by the presence of Fc receptors (see Chapter 1). Thus, 'damaged' platelets are removed from the circulation to the RE system in the spleen.

SUGGESTED FURTHER READING

Beckers, E.A.M., van Gulder, C., Overbeeke, M.A.M. and van Rhenen, D.J. (2001) Intravascular hemolysis by IgA red cell antibodies. *The Netherlands Journal of Medicine* **58**, 204–208.

British Committee for Standards in Haematology Haemostasis and Thrombosis Taskforce: www.bcshguidelines.com

Hoffbrand, A.V., Moss, P.A.H. and Pettit, J.E. (2006) *Essential Haematology*, 5th edn. Oxford: Blackwell Science.

Pallister, C. (2008) *Haematology*, 2nd edition. Oxford: Scion Publishing Ltd.

Semple J.W. and Freedman, J. (2006) Mechanisms underlying autoimmunity in hematology. *Drug Discovery Today: Disease Mechanisms* **3**, 231–235.

SELF-ASSESSMENT QUESTIONS

1. Define warm haemolytic anaemia and give examples of diseases in which it may occur.

2. List the likely causes of cold haemolytic anaemia.
3. Describe the mechanisms of red cell destruction in haemolytic anaemia.
4. Differentiate among the mechanisms of drug-induced haemolytic anaemia.
5. Describe the changes in the blood leading to kernicterus and how it may be prevented.
6. List the occasions when prophylactic anti-D immunoglobulin should be given to the mother.
7. Explain the principle of the Kleihauer–Betke test.
8. Describe the three situations in which antibody production can affect platelets.
9. Define the term 'purpura'.

Blood products and components

Learning objectives
After studying this chapter you should be able to:

■ List the components derived from blood

■ Describe the physiological role of each component

■ Discuss the processing and use of components derived from plasma

■ Describe the storage of blood products

■ Describe the clinical use of blood products

■ Discuss the importance of quality control procedures

9.1 INTRODUCTION TO BLOOD COMPONENTS

The most effective way to make optimum use of donated blood is to separate it into its various components. The patient can then be transfused with the component in which they are deficient. This strategy results in a wider availability of blood products and components and has the advantage that the patient is exposed to fewer transfusion-related risks. This chapter will describe the products available, the production process and clinical use, and the procedures developed to prevent blood-transmitted infections.

The physiological role of blood is to provide volume for circulation and the transport of many substances and cellular elements. By cellular elements we mean the blood cells – red cells (erythrocytes), white cells (leucocytes) and platelets (thrombocytes). The volume is made up by plasma, which contains proteins such as fibrinogen, albumin and globulin (including the immunoglobulins). These large molecules provide the plasma with **colloid osmotic pressure** (see *Box 9.1*).

In addition, the plasma contains the coagulation factors. From a transfusion aspect, these are the essential components of plasma which may be transfused to a patient in need of a particular component. *Table 9.1* lists the products and components available from whole blood for transfusion to a patient. The clinical requirements of a patient are important in deciding

---

Box 9.1 Colloid osmotic pressure

Colloid osmotic activity is largely provided for in the blood by the physiological concentration of albumin, which accounts for 60–80% of the normal colloid osmotic pressure of plasma. The dynamic between circulating blood and extracellular fluid levels in the tissues was described by Starling in 1896. His work showed that the plasma proteins had oncotic activity, meaning that colloid solutions were able to remain in the blood vessels rather than diffuse into the tissues. This is of particular importance when the capillaries and tissues are damaged such as in a burns patient. By transfusing a colloid solution such as albumin, the circulating volume can be maintained and transport can occur effectively. A state known as haemorrhagic shock results if the circulating volume is insufficient, i.e. the patient is hypovolaemic. Tissues become ischaemic, i.e. starved of oxygen, and tissue damage, or necrosis, occurs.

Table 9.1 Products and components from donor blood

Components available from whole blood	Products derived from pooled plasma
Red cell concentrates	Human albumin solution
Platelet concentrates	Immunoglobulins
Fresh frozen plasma	Coagulation factor concentrates
Cryoprecipitate	Prothrombin complex concentrate
Leucodepleted red cells in CPDA	
Leucodepleted SAG-M red cells	

which blood product should be transfused. A patient who has sustained a **massive blood loss**, for example following surgical or obstetric haemorrhage or a road traffic accident, has two major requirements: to replace the lost volume and to provide oxygen-carrying capacity. Blood volume may be replaced by a number of fluids, e.g. human albumin solution, saline, colloid solutions or whole blood. Oxygen-carrying capacity is provided by red blood cells so the patient may be given whole blood or a red cell concentrate. There are few clinical situations for which whole blood is the component of choice; most units of donor blood are separated into components. Massive blood loss would also need replacement of coagulation factors which have been lost during haemorrhage. Fresh frozen plasma is a blood product containing high levels of coagulation factors and is described later in this chapter.

Another clinical transfusion requirement is pre- and post-surgical procedures. Prior to a surgical operation, the patient's haemoglobin level, red cell count and **haematocrit** are measured by the laboratory to ensure that these parameters are within normal limits as there will be further blood loss during surgery (see *Box 9.2*).

A 'top up' of red cell concentrate (also known as packed red cells) may be needed (see *Colour plate 3a*). Similar parameters are checked post-surgery

> **Box 9.2 The haematocrit**
>
> The haematocrit (Hct) is a ratio obtained by measuring the volume of plasma and the volume of packed red blood cells after the unit or patient sample of blood has been centrifuged. It is sometimes called the packed cell volume, or PCV. The mean value for males is 0.47 and for females is 0.42 (expressed as a ratio per litre of plasma to litre of red cells). It is much higher in neonates due to the increased haemoglobin levels at birth. A unit of donated blood may have the haematocrit checked to ensure it is adequate for transfusion to a patient.

and further transfusion of red cells may be required, as well as coagulation factors either in the form of fresh frozen plasma or as specific clotting factors. There are many haematological examples in which a patient may suffer from **anaemia** in the absence of haemorrhage. These include deficiencies of dietary components such as iron, vitamin B12 or folic acid, or genetic disorders in which haemoglobin synthesis is ineffective, for example thalassaemia. Disorders affecting the bone marrow, such as leukaemia and aplastic anaemia, result in ineffective haemopoiesis and leucopoiesis. Furthermore, the treatment for these disorders can prevent normal bone marrow activity, resulting in anaemia or a low platelet count. In these cases, much support therapy is required from blood products, especially red cell concentrates, platelet concentrates and coagulation factors.

9.2 BLOOD COMPONENTS FOR TRANSFUSION

Blood components and products are provided by voluntary donors and processed by the National Blood Service in the UK. About 4500 donors per week are sourced at each UK Blood Centre. A donated 'unit' consists of approximately 450–500 ml of blood mixed with anticoagulant. An alternative process for the collection of blood components is that of **apheresis**, which uses cell separation equipment and centrifugation. It is particularly used to separate plasma or platelets, returning the remaining red cells to the donor in the same process (see 'Platelet concentrates' in Section 9.4 below). The selection of donors is a careful process governed by a variety of factors which aim to provide for the safety of both the donor and the recipient (see Chapter 11). The processing, storage and clinical use of donor blood and its components will be described.

Red cell concentrates

Red cell concentrates are obtained from individual units of donor blood by centrifugation and removal of the plasma. The volume of plasma removed will determine the haematocrit of the product. If the haematocrit is high, then the blood is more viscous and may cause problems in transfusion, particularly if given to neonates or the elderly. Red cells contain the oxygen-carrying molecule haemoglobin (Hb). The balance between the portion of oxygen circulating bound to Hb and the portion released to the tissues is regulated by the metabolite 2,3-diphosphoglycerate (2,3-DPG), which is present in almost equimolar amounts in the red cells. It acts by lowering the affinity of Hb for oxygen at the concentration normally present in red cells. Thus, oxygen is released to the tissues as blood circulates in the capillary bed. The anticoagulant into which the donor blood is taken must ensure that sufficient quantities of 2,3-DPG are maintained for the length of time that the blood may be used for transfusion. A solution of **citrate, phosphate, dextrose-adenine** (**CPDA**) is normally used for anticoagulation and preservation. It is used to prevent the donor blood from clotting. Adenine is required to maintain adenine diphosphate levels, which allows the red cells to continue to be metabolically active whilst in storage. Citrate is commonly used for its anticoagulant properties as it removes calcium ions which are required for the coagulation factors to form a clot. See *Box 9.3* for an explanation of plasma and serum.

Box 9.3 The difference between plasma and serum

The terms 'plasma' and 'serum' are often used interchangeably in laboratories. However, their components differ and it is important when testing blood to know which is required. The difference is due to the clotting protein, fibrinogen. Fibrinogen is converted to fibrin strands in the process of clot formation. Blood naturally clots if taken from the body and left to stand for a period of time. The result is a separation of serum, which is fibrinogen free, and a clot consisting of red cells. As the clot is semi-solid, clearly this could not be allowed to happen in blood intended for transfusion. Thus, the addition of an anticoagulant substance, e.g. citrate, prevents the clotting process. Blood which has been anticoagulated consists of plasma (containing fibrinogen) and free red cells.

The expiry period for red cell concentrates, stored at 2–6°C, is 35–42 days. As the blood ages, the 2,3-DPG levels and, therefore, the oxygen-carrying capacity, are reduced. A combination of preservative substances may be added to the red cells to prolong metabolic activity and levels of 2,3-DPG. This is called an 'additive solution' and consists of saline containing adenine, glucose and mannitol, called **SAGM**. Red cells with SAGM added are also less viscous and therefore easier and quicker to transfuse (see *Box 9.4*).

Box 9.4 Additive solutions for donor blood

The additive solution SAGM is commonly used in the UK. It consists of: sodium chloride (140 mmol l^{-1}) as a diluent of physiological concentration, adenine (1.5 mmol l^{-1}), glucose (50 mmol l^{-1}) and mannitol (30 mmol l^{-1}). This solution maintains the ATP levels required for red cell metabolism and prevents haemolysis of red cells.

The use of SAGM prolongs the shelf life of blood and allows most of the plasma to be removed. This means that more plasma can be made available for fractionation into products. The Hct of SAGM red cells ranges between 50 and 70%. However, as most of the plasma proteins have been removed, the viscosity is reduced.

Table 9.2 Normal values of blood parameters

Parameter	Male	Female	Both genders	Neonates
Hb (g l⁻¹)	135–175	115–155		140–200
Platelets (× 10^9 l⁻¹)			150–400	
Red cells (×10^9 l⁻¹)	4.5–6.5	3.9–5.6		
Haematocrit (%)	40–52	36–48		
Fibrinogen (g l⁻¹)			1.75–4.5	1.5–3.0

A rise of approximately $10 \, g \, l^{-1}$ of haemoglobin should be seen in the patient for each transfused unit of red cells. Some normal ranges for blood parameters are shown in *Table 9.2*. All red cell products are selected specifically for patients to prevent blood group incompatibility or infusion of foreign antigens into a patient. Over 600 red cell antigens have been discovered; however, it is essential to exclude the presence of antigens which, if transfused, may result in the formation of **clinically significant** antibodies, that is, those antibodies which lead to a patient having a transfusion reaction. See Chapters 5, 6 and 7 for details of antigens and antibodies in blood groups. The methods available for blood compatibility testing are described fully in Chapter 10.

Leucocyte-depleted blood components

The risk of transmission of variant Creutzfeldt–Jakob disease (vCJD) via donor blood transfusion has had a major impact on the processing of donor blood in the UK. The process of leucodepletion is used for all donor units in the UK and in many other countries in Europe. This process became mandatory in the UK in an attempt to reduce the unknown risk of prion transmission by leucocytes (see Chapter 11). In addition, leucocytes transmit viruses, express HLA antigens (see Chapter 12) and produce cytokines. For these reasons, they may cause infection, particularly with cytomegalovirus (CMV), and may cause **non-haemolytic febrile transfusion reactions**. The latter is a strong indication for the depletion of leucocytes in blood in certain patients (see Chapter 10). Leucocytes are removed from the blood by filtering through a leucocyte-specific filter prior to transfusion. The aim is to remove sufficient leucocytes from the red cell or platelet donation to prevent adverse effects and a residual level of less than 5×10^6 leucocytes per unit of red cells (or adult therapeutic dose of platelets) is considered to be satisfactory. Leucocyte-depleted products may be used as an alternative to CMV-negative products in cases where the viral transmission of CMV is to be avoided for patients at risk. Transfusion of infants below 1 year old and neonates should always be with CMV-negative blood components. This also applies to intrauterine transfusions. Transfusion support in stem cell transplant patients should also be with CMV-negative blood products as these patients are immunosuppressed.

Washed red cells

A unit of red cells may be washed in saline to remove residual plasma, leucocytes and platelets. Plasma proteins may cause reactions in patients who have IgA deficiency. Other examples are patients who are found to have allergic reactions to transfusion for no apparent reason or have developed autoimmune haemolytic anaemia. In this case, antibodies are causing haemolysis, which is enhanced by the presence of complement. These are very rare clinical disorders in which adverse reactions to transfusion may be avoided by washing the donated red cells in saline. Thus, all traces of plasma proteins are removed.

Frozen red cells

The process of freezing is used for long-term storage of red cells from donors with rare blood groups. The red cells are frozen in liquid nitrogen vapour at −80°C using a cryoprotectant, that is, a substance which prevents the formation of large ice crystals, thus allowing cell membranes to be unaffected by freezing. In this way, red cells can be stored for many years.

9.3 PLASMA-DERIVED BLOOD COMPONENTS

The separation of blood into the cellular components and plasma by centrifugation has been explained earlier. This will also occur if the blood is left to sediment naturally, although the process takes much longer. The speed of centrifugation determines whether cellular components will be present in plasma as the cells sediment according to their difference in density, size and ability to deform. This means that if the blood is centrifuged at a high relative centrifugal force (RCF), the red cells, leucocytes and platelets will eventually be forced to the lower portion, leaving a virtually cell-free plasma component. Plasma has the lowest density with a specific gravity of $1026 \, \mathrm{g \, cm^{-3}}$ at 20°C, whereas red cells have a specific gravity of $1100 \, \mathrm{g \, cm^{-3}}$. The majority of leucocytes, which are less dense than red cells, sediment at the interface between the red cells below and the plasma above. This is known as the 'buffy layer'. Careful removal of the plasma, without disturbing this layer, should result in a leucocyte- and platelet-depleted volume of plasma, known as platelet-poor plasma (PPP). Platelets are the smallest and least dense of the cellular components of the blood and therefore take the longest to sediment. If blood is centrifuged at a lower RCF, the platelets remain in the upper layer of plasma. This results in a plasma component which is 'platelet rich' (PRP), to be discussed later in this chapter.

In blood transfusion practice, the aspiration of plasma components is performed in a 'closed system' to prevent infection of the blood by exposure

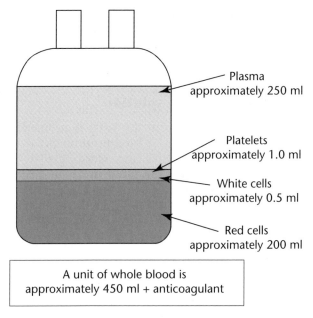

Plasma
approximately 250 ml

Platelets
approximately 1.0 ml

White cells
approximately 0.5 ml

Red cells
approximately 200 ml

A unit of whole blood is
approximately 450 ml + anticoagulant

Figure 9.1
A unit of blood after centrifugation showing the relative volumes of each component.

to the environment. The plastic containers into which the blood is taken from the donor vein are specially made with a series of 'ports' to which plastic tubing has been attached so that a number of components can be removed from the original donor unit using an aseptic technique (see *Fig. 9.1*).

Plasma fractionation

The technique of separating plasma into its components was first described by Cohn in 1944.

Box 9.5 The process of Cohn fractionation

Cohn was working at the Harvard Protein Laboratory in the USA when he developed a protein purification system that was initially used with bovine plasma. Extensive supplies of plasma had been required during World War II and albumin was thought to be the plasma protein which was most effective in providing oncotic activity. The protein purification technique was based on solid/liquid separation techniques using cold ethanol fractionation. He used a reaction medium in which the conditions, such as temperature, hydrogen ion concentration and ionic strength, were carefully controlled. Cold ethanol was added to partition the major proteins by their presence either in the precipitate or supernatant.

PPP may be pooled from large numbers of donors or used as an individual product. While the pooling of plasma has created an increase risk of viral disease transmission, the treatment of plasma using heat or chemical techniques has been largely successful in eliminating this risk. Pooled plasma is used to obtain a variety of components for treating patients. These are described in the following section.

Human albumin solution

The role of albumin in the body is primarily to provide colloid osmotic activity and to act as a binding protein for various substances including bilirubin, lipids, metallic ions and drugs.

Low levels of albumin result from the shock and trauma associated with blood loss or severe burns. Albumin was first used in World War II as an alternative to whole blood to treat the many casualties. Albumin is produced from cold ethanol fractionation using pooled plasma donations. It is filtered and heated to 60°C for 10 hours so that any viruses present are inactivated. It is then stored for 2 weeks at 30–32°C and examined for bacterial contamination. It is a safe, but expensive, plasma component with a shelf life of 2–3 years when stored between 2 and 25°C. No blood grouping is necessary when issuing this product to patients.

Immunoglobulins

Immunoglobulins are obtained either from standard blood donation or by the process of apheresis. Selected donors are tested for the presence of immunoglobulins, and, in particular, for high titres of IgG antibodies in their blood. Immunoglobulins are harvested and a specific immunoglobulin can then be administered by intravenous or intramuscular infusion into patients with immunoglobulin deficiency. A deficiency of IgG may be inherited or secondary to disease or drug treatments. A rare example of immunoglobulin depletion is severe combined immunodeficiency syndrome. In addition, intravenous immunoglobulin may be used as prophylaxis for a number of infectious diseases including tetanus, hepatitis B and CMV. Immunoglobulins can be stored for up to 12 months at 4–6°C. The prophylactic anti-D immunoglobulin given to Rh D-negative mothers is also provided; however, there is increasing interest in antibody-producing recombinant cell lines for the supply of immunoglobulins.

Coagulation factor concentrates

It is necessary to understand the process of **haemostasis**, which literally means 'to stop bleeding', so that the importance of providing coagulation factor concentrates can be appreciated. A simplified scheme of blood coagulation is shown in *Fig. 9.2*. Factors which may be administered to treat coagulation deficiencies include factor VIII and factor IX.

Factor VIII concentrate

The clotting factor VIII is produced by the liver hepatocytes and has a role in the coagulation cascade leading to the formation of the fibrin clot. When

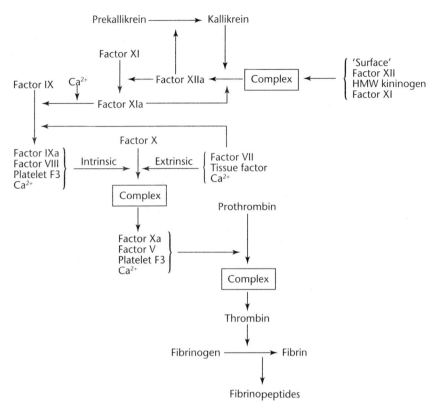

Figure 9.2
Simplified scheme of blood coagulation.

factor VIII is converted to its activated form, factor VIIIa, it allows the process to continue until fibrin is formed. In this way, haemorrhage is prevented. Clinical indications for the transfusion of factor VIII are: haemophilia A, von Willebrand disease (vWd) and acquired deficiency of factor VIII, for example due to liver disease.

Haemophilia A is a congenital deficiency of factor VIII which may be mild, moderate or severe. It results in haemorrhage, particularly into the joints, and is very painful. The factor VIII gene is found on the X chromosome and mainly affects males, though females may be carriers, or, rarely, sufferers, of the disorder. Gene mutations include premature stop codons and deletions within the 26 exons of the gene. The most severe defect occurs as a result of a mutation pattern in intron 22 in which DNA transcription is disrupted so that no functional factor VIII is formed. A similar haemorrhagic disorder, vWd, has an autosomal dominant inheritance pattern. The defect results in the inability to form von Willebrand factor (vWf), a co-factor to which factor VIII must be bound in the circulation. Without the presence of vWf, the clotting cascade cannot proceed to fibrin formation. The treatment for these disorders is to infuse factor VIII concentrate, thus restoring this factor in the blood to levels which are effective in haemostasis. The factor VIII level in the blood should be raised by approximately 2 U dl⁻¹ per unit of factor VIII infused. One of the problems of factor VIII infusion is that approximately 20% of haemophiliacs develop inhibitory antibodies (inhibitors) to human factor VIII concentrate which render it ineffective in clotting. However, other sources of factor VIII are available such as animal, especially porcine, or recombinant factor VIII. Recombinant sources of factor VIII are selected wherever possible to remove the risk of transmitting infection. Haemophiliacs were severely affected by the transmission of human immunodeficiency virus (HIV) from factor VIII concentrates in the early 1980s. This was prior to the stringent testing for viruses in blood products and many haemophiliacs became infected with HIV and hepatitis C as a result.

The process of plasma-derived factor VIII production requires plasma pooled from large numbers of donors. The inactivation of viruses is achieved during the fractionation process itself, as well as by heating to 80°C for 72 hours. Treatment with chemicals such as solvent/detergent is also possible (see *Box 9.6*).

Recombinant factor VIII is produced from commercially available cell lines, for example hamster ovary or kidney cells, which are grown in culture medium. The cells have been genetically engineered to contain the human gene for factor VIII. Factor VIII is produced as the cells are grown in culture and is then harvested, purified by chromatography and heated or chemically treated to inactivate viruses. Inhibitors to recombinant factor VIII occur in approximately 30% of patients.

Ultimately, it is likely that treatment will be available in the form of gene therapy for these disorders.

Box 9.6 Pathogen inactivation of blood products

The solvent detergent technique

The solvent detergent technique is used in the preparation of factors VIII and IX and also immunoglobulins. First, a solvent is added to the plasma which removes the lipid viral envelope. A detergent is then added which inactivates the viral contents. Both the solvent and detergent are removed by physical separation techniques in which the solvent and detergent are dissolved in oil. Column chromatography is then used to isolate factors VIII and IX.

The methylene blue technique

Methylene blue is a dye that has been found to be effective in pathogen inactivation and is used to treat fresh frozen plasma. Methylene blue binds to nucleic acids and, on illumination with white light, **singlet oxygen** is formed which destroys viral DNA and RNA. Thus, viral replication does not take place.

Psoralens

Psoralens are tricyclic organic chemicals, identified by 'S' and a number, e.g. S-59. They are found to occur in nature in fruits such as bananas and figs. However, when added to a blood product they intercalate with strands of nucleic acids and both viral and bacterial DNA are inactivated. Psoralens are particularly used for pathogen inactivation of platelet concentrates.

Other factor concentrates

Whilst most of the clotting factors are available through both plasma fractionation and recombinant DNA technology, factor VII and factor IX concentrates (which includes factors X and II, protein C and protein S) are also of clinical value. Prothrombin complex concentrate contains factors II, V and X and is available from commercial sources for patients who are bleeding due to deficiency of these factors. The clinical requirements for their use are similar to those described earlier, for example acquired coagulation factor deficiency or liver disease will result in multiple clotting deficiencies which may be treated by factor concentrates. Haemophilia B, or Christmas disease, is a congenital deficiency of factor IX and requires regular infusion of factor IX concentrate to prevent haemorrhage and bruising.

9.4 PLASMA-DERIVED PRODUCTS FROM SINGLE DONATIONS

Fresh frozen plasma (FFP) is produced from single donations of blood in which the plasma has been harvested and rapidly frozen (see *Colour plate 3b*). Fresh frozen plasma is rich in coagulation factors. Coagulation factors undergo various degrees of deterioration, especially when not kept frozen. Plasma (platelet poor) is removed from the red cells within 6 hours of the blood being donated, frozen rapidly at –70°C, and stored at –30°C to maintain the coagulation factors at optimum levels. Fresh frozen plasma is leucodepleted and may be virally inactivated using chemical treatment with methylene blue or solvent/detergent in order to ensure the safety of the product regarding disease transmission (see *Box 9.6*). Coagulation deficiencies or haemorrhage can occur in many clinical situations such as massive blood loss, infection or surgery to the liver (which is usually the site of synthesis for clotting factors), and acquired multiple coagulation factor deficiencies. Disseminated intravascular coagulation (DIC) is a clinical syndrome in which the coagulation system becomes out of control, usually due to procoagulants being released into the circulation secondary to a disease, such as cancer, or disorder (e.g. obstetric problems). Coagulation factors V and VIII, fibrinogen and platelets quickly become depleted in the presence of DIC and thus FFP can be infused to prevent further haemorrhage. It is usual for a patient to be infused with a single litre of FFP at a time and for the clinical benefit to be assessed by coagulation tests in the laboratory. Recipients of FFP should be given ABO group specific or AB donated plasma to prevent a transfusion reaction due to anti-A or anti-B (see *Table 9.3*). Once FFP has been thawed for use, it should be stored at 2–6°C and infused within 24 hours. The coagulation factors are labile proteins and the levels of factor VIII and factor V in particular fall quickly after thawing.

The clinical case of severe haemorrhage is used below (see *Box 9.7*) to exemplify the use of the blood products described above.

Table 9.3 Fresh frozen plasma selection by blood group

Recipient's group	O	A	B	AB
1st choice	O*	A	B	AB
2nd choice	A	AB	AB	A
3rd choice	B	B	A	B
4th choice	AB	–	–	–

Notes:

*Group O FFP must only be given to group O recipients.

Group A and B must be negative for high-titre ABO antibodies; AB plasma is haemolysin-free and suitable for any blood group but is often in short supply.

FFP is not antigenic for RhD so Rh D-positive FFP can be given to either RhD-positive or -negative patients. There is no requirement for prophylactic anti-D.

Box 9.7 The management of massive transfusion

In situations where a patient has lost a large amount of blood, massive transfusion of blood products is required to save life. Massive transfusion is defined as 'the replacement of a patient's total blood volume by allogeneic stored blood', usually within a period of 24 hours (Isaac & Hamilton, 2006).

This event usually occurs due to a medical emergency such as a road accident, intensive care treatment post-surgery, in the operating theatre or in obstetric cases. The result of overwhelming haemorrhage is acute hypovolaemic shock. The patient exhibits the symptoms of low blood pressure and extensive tissue damage will follow.

The priorities in massive transfusion are to replace and maintain the blood volume, to maintain haemostasis, i.e. coagulation factors and platelets, and to optimize the oxygen-carrying capacity by maintaining the haematocrit at >0.24 and haemoglobin levels above 80 g l^{-1}. In addition, it is needed to correct metabolic disturbances such as hypocalcaemia, hyperkalaemia, acid base disturbance and hypothermia and to maintain plasma colloid osmotic pressure.

The laboratory management of massive transfusion is as follows:

- blood sample for ABO and Rh group
- haemoglobin concentration
- haematocrit
- coagulation profile, e.g. prothrombin time
- tests of renal function, e.g. urea and electrolytes

A number of blood products may be used for transfusion support. For example, FPP should be given to replace coagulation factors, which are labile in stored blood, and platelet concentrate given to supplement platelets. These should be transfused when blood loss and fluid replacement have reached approximately 40% of total volume. The decision regarding whether, and how much, FFP should be used for treating a patient with major blood loss should be guided by timely tests of coagulation (including near-patient tests). 'Formulae' to guide replacement strategies should not be used.

Cryoprecipitate

Cryoprecipitate is a source of factor VIII extracted from the plasma of single donors. In previous years, it was used extensively for the treatment of haemophiliacs but is now less often used, as viral-inactivated factor VIII concentrate is widely available. Cryoprecipitate was discovered in 1965 and is formed, as the name suggests, by the precipitation of a fraction of the plasma which is enriched with factor VIII when frozen and then slowly thawed. In this process, FFP is thawed gradually at 4°C and then stored at −30°C. The plasma must be frozen within a few hours of blood collection as factor VIII has a short half-life at room temperature. Cryoprecipitate is mainly used as a source of factor VIII and fibrinogen to treat DIC and is sometimes used in patients with low plasma levels of this protein.

Platelet concentrates

Platelets are normally formed in the bone marrow and released into the circulation where they have a role in haemostasis. Platelets clump together, or aggregate, in response to substances produced when the blood vessel lining has been damaged. A platelet plug is formed, which has the effect of preventing blood loss from the damaged vessel wall. The coagulation system is also activated to form fibrin and a platelet–fibrin thrombus results. Patients who are lacking in platelets are therefore prone to bruising due to small haemorrhages into the tissues, and bleeding, for example nose bleeds (epistaxis). This condition is known as **thrombocytopenia**. Low numbers of circulating platelets may be due to a disease, particularly leukaemia and aplastic anaemia. Drug treatment such as the use of cytotoxic drugs which affect the haemopoietic cells in the bone marrow may result in thrombocytopenia, while haemopoietic stem cell transplant patients may also suffer from this condition. Patients requiring massive transfusion or heart–lung bypass surgery are likely to have a low circulating platelet count due to dilution. Inherited disorders of platelet function are sometimes detected and these patients require platelet transfusions to prevent haemorrhage.

The transfusion of platelet concentrates is an effective way of raising the circulating platelet numbers (see *Colour plate 3c*). The normal platelet count for adults and children is 150–400 × 10^9 l^{-1}; levels may fall to as low as <5 × 10^9 l^{-1} and a number of units of platelet concentrate may be required to raise the levels to ⩾20 × 10^9 l^{-1} in order to control haemorrhage. The effectiveness is established in the laboratory by checking the platelet count pre- and post-transfusion. While the normal survival of platelets is approximately 10 days, this is reduced in transfused platelets to 4 days. Thus, regular transfusions may be needed. The infusion of a single adult dose of platelets consists of approximately 2.5–3 × 10^{11} platelets.

Platelet concentrates are prepared by one of two methods. First, donated blood is subjected to a slow centrifugation in which the platelets, having a relatively low density, settle in the upper plasma layer. The platelet-rich plasma is then aspirated into a 'satellite' plastic pack and further centrifuged to sediment the platelets into a concentrate in a small volume of plasma. Four of these are then pooled to provide one adult dose. The upper layer of PPP is aspirated and used for further fractionation. The second method is by **plasmapheresis** using a cell separator. This technique involves the removal of donor blood by insertion of a catheter into a vein; as the blood enters the cell separator, selective centrifugation takes place at a speed which removes the platelets. The remaining platelet-depleted blood is returned to the donor via a catheter inserted into a vein in the other arm. This method results in a higher yield of platelets (at least 3.0×10^{11} l^{-1} compared with 5.5×10^{10} l^{-1} by the whole blood donor method). The process of leucodepletion using filtration is also included. Whichever technique is used, the subsequent conditions in which the platelets are kept prior to transfusion are important. The physiological role of platelets is to become activated in response to trauma and this must be prevented during storage so that the platelets can still be effective in platelet plug formation once they are transfused. Thus, platelets are stored in incubators at temperatures between 20 and 24°C, with continuous gentle movement provided by placing on an 'agitator'. Gas-permeable plastic bags are used for the preparation and storage of platelet concentrates. Continuous agitation allows gas exchange to take place through the bag. This prevents platelet metabolism becoming anaerobic, the result of which would be a build up of lactate causing a drop in pH which then causes the platelets to aggregate.

The shelf-life of platelets is currently 5 days. They may be irradiated if the patient's condition requires (see 'Leucocyte-depleted blood components' in Section 9.2 above). Platelets for newborn infants may be prepared using the technique of apheresis as well as single donor sources. The donated platelets can then be split into four smaller units for transfusion to the infant. Further procedures are also required for neonates, including selecting from CMV-negative donors and screening extensively to exclude the presence of antibodies. Contamination of platelets with bacteria is a concern due to the storage temperature, and this is currently one of the most frequent transfusion-transmitted risks (see Chapter 11). If the platelet packs look cloudy or turbid, then they should not be transfused. Screening platelets for bacterial contamination by semi-automated techniques are currently being trialled in the UK. Blood group-specific requirements for the selection of platelets are shown in *Table 9.4.*

Table 9.4   Selection of platelet concentrate by blood group

Recipient's group	O+	O–	A+	A–	B+	B–	AB+	AB–
1st choice	O+	O–	A+	A–	B+	B–	AB+	AB–
2nd choice	O–	O+	A–	A+	B–	B+	A+	A–
3rd choice	A+	A–	B+	B–	A+	A–	A–	A+

Note:

Rh D-negative females must be given Rh D-negative platelets if possible. If Rh D-positive platelets are transfused, it is important to also inject prophylactic anti-D (see Chapter 8).

9.5 QUALITY ASSURANCE PROCEDURES FOR BLOOD AND BLOOD PRODUCTS

All products derived from blood are subjected to rigorous quality control procedures by Blood Centres and the Bio-Products Laboratory in the UK. Component processing must comply with the regulations and standards of Good Manufacturing Practice and Good Pharmaceutical Practice as appropriate. It is necessary to ensure that the product contains adequate levels of the component stated on its label, and also that it is processed and stored correctly from manufacture to the issuing of the products to the hospital and finally to the patient at the bedside. The prevention of disease transmission by blood components is highly significant, particularly since the emergence of HIV and more recently the reported cases of the transmission of vCJD by transfusion of blood from affected donors. Further discussion of disease transmission by blood products and components can be found in Chapter 11. Blood safety regulations require that all serious adverse events or reactions in both the UK and EU are reported to a body known as the Medicines and Healthcare Products Regulatory Agency (MHRA). The role of this body is to enforce the standards laid down by the EU Blood Directive. Hospital-based blood banks must demonstrate that they are complying with the safety standards. This involves meticulous documentation of processes, procedures and events or incidents which may develop in a transfused patient. One example of this is the traceability of a blood product. It must be possible to 'tag' a unit of blood or blood product and follow its journey from the arm of the donor to the hospital and thence to the patient. Units of blood are selected for compatibility with individual patients, but are not always required to be transfused. They may then be reselected for another patient, and occasionally even reach their expiry date without being transfused and so must be discarded from the pool of blood stocks, though this wastage is avoided wherever possible. Transfused patients may leave hospital and continue with life for some years before developing symptoms of a disease which has resulted from the transfusion. These occasions are very rare but it is crucial to be able to trace the identity of the donor or donors. The use of bar codes on all blood components has been invaluable, while the computerization of blood stocks has reduced the source of human error. The labelling of a unit of blood/blood product provides much detail of information in this form, including the blood group, the expiry date, the unique identifying number of the donor, the blood centre of issue and the type of product.

The Serious Adverse Blood Reactions and Events (SABRE) is an online reporting system in the UK which facilitates the reporting from hospitals of any incidents which may be of concern. The Serious Hazards of Transfusion (SHOT) scheme is a voluntary UK scheme which collects and reports on data for adverse events in transfusion and is more fully described in Chapter 11.

SUGGESTED FURTHER READING

British Committee for Standards in Haematology Haemostasis and Thrombosis
Taskforce: www.bcshguidelines.com

Council of Europe Expert committee (2001) Pathogen inactivation of labile blood
products. *Transfusion Medicine* **11**, 149–175.

Higgins, C. (2007) Transmissability of CJD during blood transfusion. *The
Biomedical Scientist* **51**, 11–13.

Hoffbrand, A.A., Moss, P.A.H. and Pettit, J.E. (2006) *Essential Haematology*, 5th
edn. Oxford: Blackwell Publishing.

Issac, J. and Hamilton, P.J. (2006) Guidelines on the management of massive
blood loss: http://www.bcshguidelines.com/pdf/bloodloss_2006.pdf (accessed
19/07/2007).

Klein, H.G. and Anstee, D.J. (2005) *Mollison's Blood Transfusion in Clinical
Medicine*, 11th edn. Oxford: Blackwell Publishing.

McClelland, D.B.L. (ed.) (2007) *Handbook of Transfusion Medicine*, 4th edn.
London: United Kingdom Blood Services/TSO.

Murphy, M.F. and Pamphilon, D.H. (2005) *Practical Transfusion Medicine*, 2nd
edn. Oxford: Blackwell Publishing.

National Blood Authority website: http://www.blood.co.uk

UK Blood Transfusion Services (2005) *Guidelines for the Blood Transfusion
Services in the United Kingdom*, 7th edn. London: United Kingdom Blood
Services/TSO; also at http://www.transfusionguidelines.org.uk

SELF-ASSESSMENT QUESTIONS

1. List the components of blood which may be processed for transfusion.
2. Give examples of clinical cases where red cell transfusion may be
    needed.
3. Describe the optimal conditions for the storage of platelets.
4. What is the role of 2,3-diphosphoglycerate (2,3-DPG) in red cells?
5. Give reasons why the presence of leucocytes in a transfusion may be of
    risk to the patient.
6. List the methods available for the removal or inactivation of viruses in
    donated blood.
7. Describe the clinical situations requiring transfusion with FFP.
8. Why is recombinant factor VIII the treatment of choice for
    haemophilia?

Haemagglutination and blood grouping methods

Learning objectives
After studying this chapter you should be able to:

■ Describe the two stages of haemagglutination

■ Describe the forces involved in antibody binding

■ Discuss the forces involved in the formation of agglutinates

■ List the methods available for overcoming zeta potential

■ List the various ways of visualizing haemagglutination reactions

■ Describe the nature and control of the antiglobulin test

■ List the causes of false agglutination test results

■ Describe the application of molecular methods to blood transfusion

■ Describe the limitations of serological methods and molecular methods

10.1 INTRODUCTION

Red cell antigen/antibody reactions are used to determine blood groups, perform antibody screening and for compatibility testing. Traditionally the visualization of red cell antigen/antibody reactions in the laboratory is achieved by either haemagglutination (or its inhibition) or haemolysis of red cells.

Haemagglutination techniques developed over many years have proved to be robust and deceptively simple to perform. The physico-chemical factors involved in agglutination, however, are much more complex. Transfusion scientists need to have a thorough understanding of the factors involved in haemagglutination in order to be able to appreciate fully how variations in reaction conditions can affect test results. A comprehensive understanding of the processes involved enables the transfusion scientist to make informed judgements on new or variant methodologies. Experience is also required to differentiate true agglutination from other phenomena which may cause 'clumping' of red cells, e.g. fibrin clots, rouleaux, comets and red cell adherence to dust and dirt (see *Box 10.1*).

Increasingly, transfusion scientists are making use of established and emerging molecular methods for typing donors and patients using DNA. Some of these methods and their application in blood transfusion are considered in Chapter 13.

Box 10.1 Phenomena which may be falsely interpreted as agglutination in slide and tube tests

Clots
Small blood clots involving red cells may be mis-read as agglutination. They usually have smooth edges, whereas agglutinates are ragged and irregular.

Rouleaux
This is the aggregation of red cells by their flat surfaces such that they resemble piles of coins. They tend to be more regular in appearance than agglutinates and, under the microscope, usually refract light differently such that they appear more orange in colour whereas agglutinates are dark. Rouleaux can often be dispersed by the addition of a drop of clean saline to the slide.

Comets
Certain high-protein techniques, such as those using albumin, cause red cells to stick together loosely. This can be differentiated from agglutination by the smooth edges and the observation that, when looking at a moving field, the sticky mass of red cells rolls along leaving a trail of free cells. In this way, it resembles a comet with a tail.

Debris
The irregular appearance of red cells adhering to debris on a slide may resemble true agglutination. By observing a moving field, the debris can usually be seen to be floating on the surface of the sample rather than within the sample as is the case with agglutination.

10.2 HAEMAGGLUTINATION

Haemagglutination occurs in two stages. In the first stage, red cell antibodies attach to their corresponding antigen. Various terms have been used to describe this stage; these include binding, sensitization, association and coating.

In the second stage, intercellular bridges are formed as the free combining sites on the red cell-attached antibodies bind to free antigen sites on adjacent red cells. The lattice thus formed is termed an agglutinate (see *Fig. 10.1*).

First stage of agglutination (binding of antibody)

The antibody-combining sites of immunoglobulins (Fab) are complementary in shape and charge to the antigens with which they react, enabling them to come into close contact and allowing the formation of reversible bonds (see Chapter 2). Several forces and types of bond are involved in this process of antibody binding.

Ionic bonds. These are formed by the transfer of electrons from donor to acceptor ionic and non-ionic groups between the antibody and its antigen.

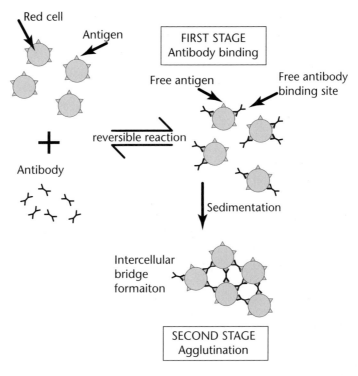

Figure 10.1
The first and second stages of haemagglutination.

This electrostatic force of attraction is inversely proportional to the square of the distance separating the charged surfaces of the red cells and antibodies. This results in a rapid increase in the magnitude of the force as the antigen and antibody surfaces approach one another. The level of ionization and charge on the antigen and antibody depend significantly on the pH of the immediate environment.

Hydrophobic bonds. These bonds arise from the tendency of non-polar groups to avoid water and adhere to one another. The amino acids alanine, leucine, isoleucine, phenylalanine and tryptophan all provide free non-polar groups for hydrophobic bonding in most protein molecules.

Hydrogen bonds. These arise from the reaction between hydrogen atoms which are covalently bound to strongly electronegative atoms (such as oxygen and nitrogen) and unshared electron pairs of other electronegative atoms. This is due to the relative electropositivity of the hydrogen nucleus. Hydrogen bonding is primarily exothermic in nature and so is further driven by reduced temperatures. This is known as Le Chatelier's principle.

Van der Waals forces. Forces that develop from the movement of electrons which produce a general attraction of molecules at short distance. The pull increases with increasing mass of the reactive sites and is inversely proportional to the seventh power of the distance separating the surfaces. This means that the antigen and antibody surfaces must come into close contact for these forces to be significant in antigen/antibody binding.

Randomization of water. This occurs as water is squeezed out when antigen and antibody surfaces come together. This causes an increase in entropy, reduces competition with hydrogen bonds, lowers the dielectric constant around polar sites and increases the attractive free energy. These are all factors which favour the binding of antigen and antibody.

Antigen/antibody reactions are dependent on both thermal (enthalpy) and disorder (entropy) factors. As the antigen/antibody complexes approach equilibrium, entropy is maximized. In addition, ionic bonds, hydrophobic bonds, hydrogen bonds and Van der Waals forces affect all reactions to some extent. Thus, the final antigen/antibody bond results from numerous types of physical force, as well as complementarity of shape and charge.

The bonds formed between antigens and antibodies are reversible and may be expressed in a mass-action relationship. See Chapter 2 for a discussion of the binding affinity of antibodies.

Being a reversible thermodynamic reaction, this binding of antibody to antigen is affected by several factors including temperature, pH, ionic strength, and the concentrations of antigen and antibody. Each of these is discussed below.

Temperature. A reduction in the reaction temperature reduces the rate of antibody association and disassociation but not necessarily the equilibrium affinity constant K, which in some cases may be increased at lower temperatures. Increases in temperature increase the rates of association and disassociation, but eventually a temperature will be reached where antibody is disassociating rather than associating, i.e. K is reduced. Those antibodies which react best at lower temperatures, such as ABO and P1 antibodies, probably depend to a larger extent on exothermic hydrogen bonds for much of their strength of attachment.

pH. The optimum range for antibody/antigen reactions is usually quoted as between pH 6.5 and 6.8 with little effect on binding noted over the range pH 5.5 to 8.5. Some anti-D antibodies show reduced binding at higher pH and some anti-M antibodies show increased binding at lower pH. Generally, a reduction in pH increases the complementarity of charges between antigen and antibody. This pH effect refers to the pH of the final reaction mixture, not the pH of individual reactants. The student's attention is drawn to the common practice of washing and suspending red cells in phosphate buffer solution with a pH of around 6.8 to 7.2. Apart from not being the optimum pH range for antibody/antigen reactions, it may be unnecessary due to the fact that both plasma and red cells act as very efficient buffers.

Ionic strength. Physiological 'normal' saline used in blood group serology is a 0.85–0.90% solution of sodium chloride in water, with an ionic strength of 0.15 mol l^{-1}. Reduction in the ionic strength of the reaction medium (typically to 0.09 mol l^{-1}) increases the rate at which the antibody binds to the antigen, but not necessarily the amount bound at equilibrium. In normal saline the mobility of individual ions is restricted by the presence of so many other ions. In low ionic strength solutions (LISS), ions are more mobile and this favours ionic bonding between antigen and antibody. In addition, the ionized groups on antigens and antibodies in saline are partially neutralized by all the free ions in the solution, thus interfering with antigen/antibody binding. In LISS, this neutralization effect is much reduced. Reducing the ionic strength of the reaction medium by too great a factor, however, facilitates the aggregation of normal serum globulins and their non-specific adhesion to red cells. This may lead to the activation and fixing of complement to the red cell. Subsequent washing of the red cells removes the globulins but complement may stay attached to the cell, leading to a false positive reaction if the cells are tested with an anti-complement-containing reagent such as polyspecific anti-human globulin reagent (see later).

Antigen and antibody concentration. An increase in the concentration of reactants favours the association reaction in the first stage of agglutination. However, this increase may reduce resultant agglutinate formation in the second stage and therefore its detection in the laboratory (see below). There is a delicate balance in the relative concentrations of antigen and antibody which needs to be achieved for optimal agglutination.

Box 10.2 Scale

To help visualize the relative differences in size between antibody molecules and red cells, consider this comparison: if a red cell was 1 m in diameter then the maximum distance between binding sites for an IgM molecule would be approximately 4 mm and for an IgG molecule approximately 1.5 mm.

Second stage of agglutination (intercellular bridge formation)

This stage involves the formation of intercellular bridges between free binding sites on red cell-bound antibodies and free antigen sites on adjacent red cells. There are three major factors affecting this stage: the forces of aggregation, the forces of repulsion and the relative concentrations of antigen and antibody. Readers also need to appreciate the relatively vast differences in size between red cells and antibody molecules (see *Box 10.2*) when considering this stage.

Aggregating forces

Every surface has a certain amount of associated energy (e.g. X ergs cm^{-2}). When aggregation or agglutination of red cells takes place, two surfaces, each of a specific surface area, for example A cm^2, come into contact. The amount of energy contained by these two surfaces, 2AX ergs, is also lost. The Second Law of Thermodynamics states that a system is in equilibrium when its free energy is at a minimum. Thus, the red cell surface tension acts in such a way as to produce aggregation and reduce surface energy.

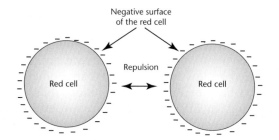

Figure 10.2
The mutual repulsion between electronegative red cells.

Repulsive forces

The most important force which opposes the aggregating effects of surface tension results from the electronegative charge of the red cell membrane. This charge arises largely from the ionization of carboxyl groups of surface sialic acid residues. The red cell surface potential charge is approximately −34 mV. As each red cell is equally charged, both in sign and magnitude (see *Fig. 10.2*), there exists between them a repulsive force which is inversely proportional to the square of the distance separating them (Coulomb's Law). It is this repulsive force which prevents red cells adhering to vessel walls or to one another. The repulsive force exerted when the flatter surfaces of two red cells come together can be ten times greater than when two curved surfaces come together. Thus, highly curved surfaces can approach each other much more closely than flat surfaces.

In the presence of an electrolyte, such as sodium (or potassium) ions in plasma or saline, each red cell is surrounded by a cloud of oppositely charged ions, that is, cations. The cloud decreases in density with increasing distance from the red cell surface. Part of this cloud of cations moves with the red cell and forms part of its kinetic unit. The line of demarcation separating the cations which move with the red cell from the remaining cations in the medium is known as the **slipping plane** (see *Fig. 10.3*).

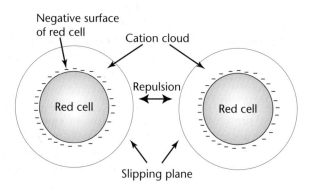

Figure 10.3
Red cells suspended in saline. Each red cell is surrounded by a cloud of cations (Na$^+$).

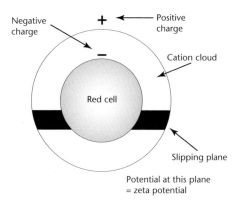

Figure 10.4
Red cells surrounded by cations represented as two concentric spheres. The inner sphere represents the electronegative surface of the red cell. The outer sphere represents the slipping plane of the electropositive cation cloud. The sum of the electrical potentials related to these two surfaces determines the total voltage that acts through the space between the two spheres and appears as the potential at the surface of the outer sphere. This is the zeta potential.

It is convenient to consider this system as analogous to the charges on two concentric spheres (see *Fig. 10.4*). The inner sphere corresponds to the red cell surface and the outer represents the slipping plane of the cation cloud. The net charge density of the cation cloud is greater than that at the red cell surface. The sum of the electrical potentials related to these two charged surfaces determines the total voltage that acts through the space between the two spheres and appears as the potential at the surface of the outer sphere. It follows that the force of repulsion between two red cells is not dependent on the value of the charge or potential at the red cell surface, but rather on the potential that exists at the boundary which marks the slipping plane. This potential is known as the **zeta potential**. Its magnitude depends on the volume net charge density of the surrounding cations, that is, the ionic strength of the medium.

The zeta potential for red cells suspended in normal saline is approximately −18 mV. At this value, the repulsive forces keep the red cells apart by approximately 18–20 nm. In order for an antibody to bring about direct agglutination of saline-suspended cells (sometimes called a **complete antibody**), it would have to span the 20 nm gap between adjacent cells. IgM antibodies have a maximum distance between binding sites of around 30 nm and so can readily span the gap between red cells. IgG antibodies have a maximum distance between binding sites of around 12 nm and so usually do not directly agglutinate red cells suspended in saline. Thus, IgG antibodies are sometimes known as **incomplete antibodies**; see *Fig. 10.5*).

However, if the antigen protrudes some distance from the cell surface, even IgG antibodies may be able to effect direct agglutination, as the distance between their target antigens would be less than the distance between the red cell surfaces. For example, ABO antigens may protrude from

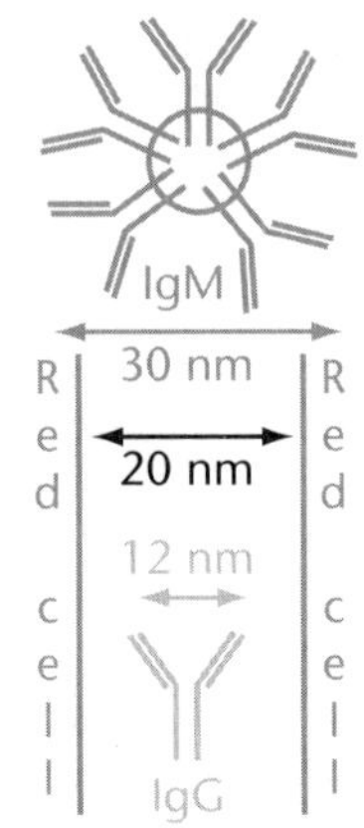

Figure 10.5
The distance between red cells suspended in normal saline. The IgG antibody molecules are too small to span the gap between adjacent red cells (incomplete antibody), whereas the IgM antibody molecules are large enough to span the gap and bring about direct agglutination (complete antibody).

the cell surface by as much as 5 nm. Although the distance between adjacent cell surfaces is 20 nm, the distance between ABO antigens may therefore be as little as 10 nm. At this distance, IgG anti-A or anti-B would be able to attach to antigens on adjacent cells and so bring about direct agglutination.

The value of the zeta potential may be reduced in order to allow closer approach of red cells either by increasing the ionic strength or the dielectric constant of the suspending medium, or by decreasing the charge at the red cell surface.

Ionic strength. As can be seen from the formula in *Box 10.3*, an increase in ionic strength reduces the zeta potential as more cations are packed around the red cell, increasing the density of the cation cloud and neutralizing more of the red cell surface charge. As described above, increasing the ionic strength decreases the amount of antibody able to bind to antigen. This

---

Box 10.3 Zeta potential

The zeta potential for human red cells at 25°C may be represented by the following formula:

$$\text{Zeta potential} = \frac{4.27}{D \cdot \mu} + \frac{309}{D} \text{ mV},$$

where D = dielectric constant of the medium and μ = ionic strength of the medium.

Red cells have a zeta potential of approximately −34 mV, which is reduced to −18 mV when the red cells are suspended in normal saline.

The critical zeta potential for an antibody is the value above which the antibody cannot bring about direct agglutination, because the red cells are held too far apart. For IgM (complete) antibodies, this value is around −23 mV. For IgG (incomplete) antibodies, this value is around −13 mV.

inhibition of antibody binding limits the usefulness of this method for reducing zeta potential.

Students often fail to understand that **decreasing the ionic strength increases the zeta potential and thus forces red cells even further apart** than in normal saline. Another way to visualize this is that, as there are fewer ions available to neutralize the red cell surface charge, there will be greater repulsion between cells. The use of a LISS technique, then, is inappropriate for the detection of antibodies by direct agglutination and this should always be considered in laboratory tests.

Dielectric constant. This is a measure of the ability of a substance to dissipate charge. As can be seen from the formula in *Box 10.3*, an increase in dielectric constant reduces the zeta potential. Certain water-soluble polymers, such as albumin, polyvinyl pyrrolidine and dextran, raise the dielectric constant of water by an amount that is dependent upon the degree to which they become polarized and oriented in an electric field. In effect, they have areas of their molecule which can be either positively or negatively charged. Thus, unlike simple ions, they are both attracted and repelled by the red cell surface charge. They are, therefore, forced to orient or rotate in such a way that they are less randomly distributed in the medium. The energy required for this polarization is obtained from the electric field surrounding the red cell and so the zeta potential is reduced.

Red cell surface charge. Reducing the electrical charge at the red cell surface obviously reduces the repulsive forces and so allows closer approach of cells. This reduction in charge is usually brought about by using proteolytic enzymes such as papain, bromelin and ficin. These enzymes are used to remove the red cell surface proteins which express the sialic acid residues that contribute the majority of the cell's negative charge.

The use of enzymes can enhance antigen/antibody reactions in a number of other ways. The enzymes may reveal new antigens or make hidden antigen sites more accessible as surface proteins are removed from the cell. Alternatively, the enzymes may increase the mobility of protein within the red cell membrane. This allows the clustering of antigen, which in turn allows the formation of multiple, adjacent intercellular bridges, thus enhancing agglutination. Enzymes may also reduce hydration at the red cell surface, favouring antigen/antibody binding. Finally, enzymes promote the production of irregular protrusions from the red cells. These protrusions have highly curved surfaces and therefore exhibit less repulsive force, allowing red cells to come together more closely.

The surface charge may also be reduced by the binding of antibodies onto the red cell. The degree of reduction is dependent on the amount of antibody bound and the charges covered. Usually the reduction in charge and the resultant reduction in zeta potential is less than 25% of the initial value. However, if sufficient IgG antibody is bound, then an IgG antibody that would normally be incomplete might cause direct agglutination of saline suspended cells. For example, cells of the rare Rh phenotype D–– (see Chapter 6) express very large amounts of Rh D antigen and therefore bind large amounts of anti-D antibody. The red cell surface charge may be reduced to such an extent that the cells are agglutinated in saline suspension with an otherwise incomplete antibody.

As mentioned earlier, reducing the ionic strength of the reaction medium by too much facilitates the aggregation of normal serum globulins and their non-specific adhesion to red cells. This can cause a considerable reduction in surface charge and lead to non-antibody-mediated red cell aggregation, which cannot be distinguished from true agglutination.

The effect of the zeta potential may be overcome in several other ways. For example, **macromolecules** increase the dielectric constant of the reaction medium, and may facilitate agglutination by bringing about large areas of cell-to-cell contact by physical adhesion (polymer bridging) of the red cells. This allows the formation of multiple, adjacent intercellular antigen/antibody bridges. Macromolecules also reduce hydration and thus increase attractive free energy around antigen/antibody binding sites and increase the extracellular colloid osmotic pressure which may induce red cell shape changes. These shape changes may allow for larger areas of cell-to-cell contact brought about by polymer bridging.

Polycationic polymers are substances such as polybrene which express multiple electropositive regions. They can readily bring about the aggregation of electronegative particles, including red cells. They facilitate agglutination by: aggregating red cells and thus bringing them closer together, allowing the formation of intercellular antigen/antibody bridges; facilitating large areas of cell-to-cell contact via polymer bridging; reducing hydration and thus increasing attractive free energy around antigen/antibody binding sites; and inducing red cell shape changes which may allow for larger areas of cell-to-cell contact brought about by polymer bridging.

Spiculation refers to the formation of long protrusions from the red cell membrane. Such protrusions have highly curved points and so exhibit less repulsion than flat surfaces. This allows closer cell-to-cell contact. ABO antibodies, in particular, have been demonstrated to induce spiculation when binding to red cells.

Concentration of antigen and antibody

Increases in the concentration of antigen or antibody favour binding in stage one of agglutination. However, the formation of agglutinates will be inhibited if the relative concentrations of antigen to antibody are not optimized. Conditions of relative excess of antigen in a reaction mixture include the use of too strong a red cell suspension, the addition of too small a volume of serum, the addition of too large a volume of cell suspension and low levels of antibody in the serum. Under these conditions, antibodies are so thinly distributed amongst the red cells that the formation of intercellular bridges will be sparse and only involve small numbers of cells (see *Fig. 10.6*). Conditions of relative excess of antibody in a reaction mixture include the use of too weak a cell suspension, cells expressing small numbers of antigen sites, the addition of too large a volume of serum, the addition of too small a volume of cell suspension and high levels of antibody in the serum. Under

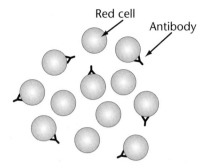

Figure 10.6
Representation of conditions of relative excess of antigen. The antibody is so sparsely distributed that few opportunities for intercellular bridge formation exist.

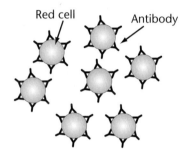

Figure 10.7
Representation of conditions of relative excess of antibody. Most antigen sites are coated with antibody so that there are too few free antigen sites available on adjacent cells for the formation of intercellular bridges.

these conditions, the majority of antigen sites are coated with antibody leaving few free antigen sites available for attachment to the free binding sites on antibodies attached to adjacent red cells. Thus, there is a reduction in intercellular bridge formation and corresponding agglutination (see *Fig. 10.7*).

10.3 METHODS

It is beyond the scope of this text to give detailed procedures for carrying out the large number of haemagglutination techniques currently available. Instead, this section gives an overview of techniques and practical considerations and relates them to the various factors involved in haemagglutination (see *Box 10.4*).

Direct agglutination

Red cells suspended in saline are kept apart, due to mutual repulsion, by a distance of approximately 20 nm. Direct agglutination of red cells suspended in saline is usually only observed with IgM antibodies, which are large enough to span the gap between adjacent cells. For this agglutination to occur, however, the correct balance of antigen and antibody concentration must be achieved. Many years of practical experience have demonstrated that most direct agglutination reactions are optimized by mixing equal volumes of serum and a 3% suspension of red cells in saline.

Direct agglutination of red cells by IgG antibodies may be brought about by using techniques which reduce the zeta potential, allowing the cells to come into closer contact. Such techniques usually have other advantages such as: encouraging multiple, intercellular antibody bridge formation by polymer bridging, antigen clustering and red cell shape changes; reducing the degree of hydration at the red cell surface, which favours antigen/antibody binding; and in the case of enzymes, making antigen sites more accessible to their corresponding antibodies. It should be remembered that techniques which allow direct agglutination by IgG antibodies may also enhance the action of IgM antibodies.

Box 10.4 Some technical factors affecting haemagglutination reactions

Reagent volumes
The volumes dispensed must be accurate and reproducible to avoid excesses of antigen or antibody. If a Pasteur or dropper pipette is being used, it must be held at the same angle for the dispensing of all reagents. A pipette held towards the horizontal relative to the test tube will dispense significantly larger volumes than a pipette held towards the vertical. Static electrical charge on the test tubes (a particular problem with plastic tubes) may affect the volume of the drop dispensed from a pipette by 'dragging' extra reagent from the tip of the pipette or by deflecting the drops as they approach the mouth of the test tube. Static may be dispersed by standing racks of tubes in a water-bath for a few seconds prior to use.

Cell concentrations
Accurate concentrations of red cell suspensions are required in order to avoid relative excesses of antigen, when the cell suspension is too strong, or antibody, when the cell suspension too weak. Most transfusion scientists learn by experience to judge commonly used cell concentrations 'by eye'.

Mixing reactants (tube and slide tests)
Thorough mixing of red cells and serum in the test tube, other than when using layering techniques, is essential to allow maximum contact between antibodies and red cells.

Zoning
A serum containing a relative excess of antibody may not bring about direct agglutination until it has been diluted to the point where optimum concentration of antigen and antibody is achieved. Further dilution of the serum leads to reducing degrees of agglutination as would normally be expected. This observation is known as zoning or the prozone effect.

Techniques which have been commonly used to bring about direct agglutination by IgG antibodies are outlined below.

Use of albumin

Usually between 20% and 30% bovine serum albumin or high molecular mass polymers are used to raise the dielectric constant of the reaction medium. This dissipates the charge surrounding the red cells, reduces the zeta potential and allows closer contact of the cells. Several variations of albumin techniques exist. These include **displacement** or **replacement** methods in which albumin is added towards the end of the reaction incubation period after the red cells have settled into a button in the tube. The high-density albumin either displaces or replaces the supernatant serum and saline to leave the cells in an albumin-rich (high dielectric constant) environment for the remainder of the incubation period. Albumin **suspension** methods, in which the red cells are suspended in an albumin solution instead of saline from the beginning of the test, are also used. Finally, **layering** methods, in which typing or test serum is layered onto a cell button at the beginning of the test, may also be employed. In this case, the serum itself provides the high-protein environment required for the test.

Albumin techniques are generally not as sensitive as some of the other techniques available for detecting IgG antibodies. In addition, there can be great variation among batches of albumin and the tests may be difficult to read due to stickiness and **comet formation** (see later). For these reasons, albumin techniques are no longer commonly used for antibody screening, although they may be useful in characterizing certain antibodies.

Use of proteolytic enzymes

Proteolytic enzymes such as papain, bromelin and ficin reduce red cell surface charge by removing proteins, particularly glycophorins, carrying electronegative sialic acid residues. Several variations are in common use, either using a one- or two-stage procedure.

In **one-stage methods**, red cells, enzyme and serum are mixed together in the same tube. There are three basic variations within this methodology. The **one-stage mix** method involves the simultaneous addition of cells, enzyme and antibody. This method has the disadvantages that the enzyme may also degrade the antibodies and some normal sera contain naturally occurring inhibitors of proteolytic enzymes. **Delay** methods, in which the red cells and enzyme are incubated together for a short time before the addition of the serum, and **inhibitor** methods, in which red cells and enzyme are incubated together for a short time and then an enzyme inhibitor is added before the addition of serum, are further examples of one-stage methods.

In **two-stage methods**, the red cells are pre-treated with enzyme, washed and then reacted with serum.

Enzyme techniques are generally very good for the detection of Rh antibodies, but as the enzymes destroy MN and Duffy antigens, such techniques cannot be used to detect antibodies in these systems. Enzyme treatment of red cells is difficult to standardize and excessive treatment can result in a large reduction in surface charge, leading to spontaneous aggregation of the cells. It is also common to find clinically insignificant auto- and pan antibodies (which react with all cells) reactive only with enzyme-treated cells. One-stage enzyme techniques have been shown to be much less reliable and less sensitive than two-stage techniques. The use of enzyme-treated cells can be a very useful tool in the characterization of a red cell antibody, but is generally no longer recommended for use as a screening technique.

Use of polycationic polymers

Polycationic polymers such as polybrene cause aggregation of electronegative red cells and so bring them into close contact. Typically, red cells and serum are incubated in a low ionic strength environment in order to accelerate antibody binding, then polybrene is added to bring the cells into close contact. The non-specific aggregation is then dispersed by the addition of sodium citrate, while any antibody-mediated agglutination remains. Polybrene techniques are rapid, good for the detection of Rh antibodies and do not suffer from the large numbers of unwanted positive results found with enzyme techniques. However, the detection rate for Kell, Duffy and Lewis antibodies can be particularly poor. For this reason, such techniques cannot be recommended for use as a stand-alone antibody screening method.

Chemical modification

The chemical modification of IgG molecules constitutes a somewhat different approach to the problem of IgG molecules being too small to bridge the gap between red cells suspended in saline. The distance between the antigen binding sites (Fab) on an IgG antibody can be increased by chemical reduction of the disulphide bonds in the hinge region. Using this technique, it has been possible to produce stable IgG antibodies capable of spanning the distance between adjacent red cells suspended in saline. This approach lends itself to the production of typing sera but has no practical application in the detection of antibodies in the sera of patients.

Indirect agglutination

The **antiglobulin test (AGT)** was described in 1945 by Coombs and coworkers and was originally called the Coombs test (see *Box 10.5*). It remains the single most important test for IgG antibody detection and identification. In the AGT, the binding of IgG antibody to red cells is visualized indirectly by the addition of **anti-human globulin (AHG) reagent**, containing antibodies to human IgG, to complete the intercellular bridging required for visible haemagglutination. The AGT may be performed directly on patients' red cells to detect *in vivo* binding of antibody (the direct antiglobulin test or **DAT**) or may be performed on cells which have been incubated with antibody *in vitro* (the indirect antiglobulin test or **IAT**). In both cases, the AHG binds to red cell-bound IgG antibodies on adjacent red cells and brings about agglutination by a red cell–antibody–AHG–antibody–red cell bridge. This intercellular bridge is much greater in size than the distance between adjacent red cells (see *Fig. 10.8*).

With direct agglutination techniques, relative excesses of antigen or antibody must be avoided in order to maximize the agglutination. This is not the case with the AGT and the ratio of antibody (serum) to antigen (cells) may be increased to allow more antibody to bind and thus increase the sensitivity of the test. Typically serum:cell ratios of 70:1 or more are used. This is double the ratio found in standard direct agglutination tests. It is the AHG reagent which brings about the eventual agglutination and

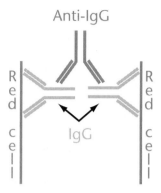

Figure 10.8
Representation of agglutination in the antiglobulin test. The red cells are too far apart for the IgG antibodies to cause direct agglutination. The addition of the anti-human globulin (AHG) reagent containing anti-IgG antibodies brings about agglutination by attaching to the red cell-bound IgG molecules and forming cell–IgG–anti-IgG–IgG–cell intercellular bridges. All free IgG must be washed away before the addition of the AHG reagent to prevent binding of the anti-IgG to free IgG rather than cell-bound IgG.

Box 10.5 The Coombs (antiglobulin) test

In the early 1940s, R.R.A. Coombs was a research worker in the Department of Pathology at Cambridge University. He became interested in the nature of incomplete Rh antibodies after a discussion over coffee one day with R.R. Race. At that time it was not known whether these incomplete antibodies were true globulin antibodies. Together they demonstrated that incomplete Rh antibody was indeed a globulin antibody. They then went on to consider a test which would more easily demonstrate these incomplete antibodies. It was in 1945, whilst travelling from London to Cambridge on a late-night, badly lit train, that Coombs first visualized the antibody on the red cell and how it might be detected using antibody to serum globulin. The basic idea for this most important of all red cell serology tests had been born.

---

this reagent must therefore be standardized to give optimal agglutination at the desired serum:cell ratio.

Most modern AHG reagents are polyspecific; that is, they contain a blend of polyclonal anti-IgG (anti-human IgG produced in animals) and a monoclonal anti-C3d (see *Box 10.6*). The anti-IgG component brings about the agglutination of IgG-coated cells as described above. The anti-C3d component is itself an IgM antibody and so brings about the direct agglutination of red cells coated with the stable complement fraction C3dg (see Chapter 3), which may be attached to red cells by the action of some clinically significant IgG or IgM antibodies. The classic AGT requires a wash phase to remove any free globulin which would otherwise neutralize the AHG reagent. IgM antibodies are particularly prone to being washed from red cells during this phase of the test and so it is more reliable to detect the complement fixed to the cell by the IgM than to try to detect the IgM antibody itself. In addition, many hundreds of molecules of complement may be fixed to the red cell by each IgM molecule, and so detecting complement is a simpler and more sensitive test.

Box 10.6 Changes in anti-human globulin reagent

Since its original use, changes have been made to the AHG reagent. The original Coombs reagent typically contained:

- Anti-IgA
- Anti-IgG
- Anti-IgM
- Antibodies to several C3 and C4 complement fragments

Modern polyspecific AHG reagents contain:

- Anti-IgG
- Anti-C3d

In attempts to increase the sensitivity of antibody detection, many workers have devised variations of the AGT. The main variations are described briefly below.

Normal ionic strength antiglobulin test (NIS-AGT)

This test is closest to the original technique in which, typically, four volumes of serum are mixed with one or two volumes of 3% red cells suspended in normal saline. The test is incubated at 37°C for 45 to 60 minutes prior to washing and addition of AHG reagent.

Low ionic strength antiglobulin test (LIS-AGT)

The use of a low ionic strength medium increases the rate of antibody uptake onto the red cells and so incubation times are reduced to between 15 and 20 minutes. Low ionic strength solutions are solutions of low salt concentration with the addition of substances to maintain isotonic conditions, such as glycine. In order to preserve the low ionic strength conditions in the test, equal volumes of serum and cells suspended in low ionic strength medium must be used. This means that, in order to achieve a more sensitive serum to cell ratio, as in the NIS-AGT, the cell concentration must be reduced to between 1.5% and 2%. Several variations of the LIS-AGT exist, including: **LIS suspension** methods, which utilize red cells suspended in a low ionic strength medium; **LIS additive** methods, which utilize the addition of an additive reagent to create the low ionic strength conditions; use of **polyethylene glycol (PEG)**, a water-soluble polymer which has been shown to act as a potentiator of antigen/antibody reactions, combined with a low ionic strength additive; and the use of the **low ionic strength polybrene** followed by washing of the red cells and the addition of AHG.

The LIS-AGT is the most common variation of the AGT in general use. As previously discussed, reducing the ionic strength can lead to the non-specific uptake of globulin and fixation of complement onto red cells, leading to false positive reactions. It is, therefore, usually recommended that LIS-AGTs are used with AHG reagents containing only anti-IgG. Many clinically insignificant antibodies which only react in LIS-AGT (and not in NIS-AGT) have been described. The detection of these antibodies can lead to delays in the provision of blood for transfusion whilst attempts are being made to identify the antibodies.

Adsorption and elution

The **adsorption of antibodies** from serum onto red cells is a procedure which may be used in a variety of situations, including the removal of unwanted antibody from a typing serum; the removal of antibody from a serum containing a mixture of antibodies, to aid identification; or to detect the presence of weakly expressed antigens by their ability to adsorb the corresponding antibody.

As previously described, increasing the concentration of antigen increases the amount of antibody bound to the red cell. In practice, this means adding a slight excess volume of concentrated red cells to a volume of serum from which the antibody is to be adsorbed.

Antibody elution is a procedure for the removal and recovery of red cell-bound antibody, into an inert medium, for subsequent identification. The inert medium containing the eluted antibody is known as the **eluate**. Examples where the preparation of an eluate is required include: the identification of antibodies bound to patients' red cells *in vivo*, as in cases of autoimmune haemolytic anaemia or haemolytic disease of the newborn; antibodies bound to transfused red cells, particularly in cases of delayed transfusion reaction; and antibodies adsorbed onto red cells from a serum containing a mixture of antibodies. In addition, antibody elution may be required to demonstrate the presence of weak antigens on red cells by the elution of the corresponding antibody from those cells after performing antibody adsorption as described above, for example in the demonstration of weak subgroups of the A antigen.

There are several elution procedures in common use. Some utilize a modification of the factors affecting the binding of antibody to antigen, such as changes in pH, temperature or ionic strength to remove the antibody. Others rely on physical disruption of the red cell membrane by solvents or freezing and thawing to release the bound antibody.

10.4 TECHNICAL CONSIDERATIONS

Antiglobulin tests

Because the AGT is the most important of all the methods available for the detection of clinically significant antibodies, the risk of false negative results in particular must be minimized. The two most common causes of a false negative AGT are inadequate washing of red cells prior to the addition of AHG and disruption of agglutinates by a poor technique for reading results.

Inadequate washing of red cells prior to the addition of AHG may leave sufficient residual serum globulin to neutralize the AHG reagent. Centrifuges used to wash cells require regular quality assurance testing to ensure that thorough washing is occurring. All negative tests should be controlled by the addition of red cells pre-sensitized with IgG antibody. If the control cells agglutinate, then sufficient free AHG is available and the negative test results are valid. If the control cells do not agglutinate, then it can be assumed that the AHG reagent has been neutralized by free serum globulin, due to inadequate washing. The negative test result in this case would be invalid and would require repeating. The pre-sensitized cells are coated in sufficient antibody to give a weak reaction with AHG. This makes them more sensitive for detecting partial neutralization of the AHG regent. Typically, the sensitized control cells should detect the presence of serum globulin at a dilution of one part in 1000.

In order to avoid false negative results due to poor reading technique, laboratories should operate an Internal Quality Assurance programme which regularly assesses an individual worker's ability to read weakly positive AGTs.

Typing red cells with a positive DAT

The red cell phenotyping of patients who have a positive DAT, for example, a patient with autoimmune haemolytic anaemia or a baby with haemolytic disease of the newborn (HDN), can pose particular problems. As the red cells from these patients are already coated in antibody, any phenotyping test which involves the use of a high-protein medium (e.g. albumin tests) or AHG may lead to a positive reaction, irrespective of whether the cell is positive or not with respect to the typing serum. To type such patients accurately it is necessary to use a direct-agglutinating, low-protein reagent such as an IgM monoclonal typing serum.

A related problem may occur when typing the red cells of a baby suffering from HDN. A false negative result may occur with a direct agglutinating typing serum if the antigen being tested for is completely masked (or blocked) by maternal antibody. For example, when attempting to Rh D type the cells from a baby with a positive DAT due to maternal anti-D, all the Rh D antigen sites on the baby's cells may already be coated with maternal antibody. They are not, therefore, available for reaction with the typing serum and the baby would type as Rh D negative. To confirm that the baby is Rh D positive, it is necessary to elute the antibody from the baby's red cells and identify it as anti-D.

Visualization of agglutination

Scoring of the strength of agglutination reactions can give valuable information about the antibody/antigen reaction. For instance, it will give clues concerning antibodies which show dosage reactions, or cells which express weaker or stronger forms of an antigen (see *Table 10.1*).

Agglutination reactions can be performed in a variety of reaction vessels, such as test tubes, slides, microplates or microtubes. They may be read macroscopically, microscopically or with the aid of a photometer or image analysis system.

Table 10.1 An example of an agglutination scoring system for tube or slide tests

Score	Agglutinates	Free cells
5+	Massive clumps	Very few
4+	Several large clumps	Some
3+	Many macroscopic clumps	More
2+	Clumps of 10–20 cells	Many
1+	Small microscopic clumps	Background of free cells
0	None	All

Reactions in test tubes. These require the red cells to be sedimented to form a button at the bottom of the tube. This is achieved either by gravity or gentle centrifugation. The cell button can then be examined for agglutination either macroscopically or microscopically. Agglutinates of red cells can be very fragile and must be handled gently. **Macroscopic examination**, which may involve the use of an optical aid such as a magnifying lens or mirror, may be achieved by resuspending the cells using a gentle **tapping** action. This method is only advisable with the most avid antibodies, such as monoclonal ABO and Rh typing sera, observing the **settling pattern and streaming** of the red cells as the tube is gently tipped. Irregular settling patterns with no streaming indicate a positive reaction, smooth settling patterns and streaming of cells on tipping indicate a negative reaction. A further method is to use the **tip and roll technique** in which the tube is gently tipped and simultaneously rolled between the thumb and first finger to resuspend the cells whilst looking for agglutination. This technique is particularly useful for reading AGTs.

Microscopic examination. Examining cell buttons for agglutination in this way is probably the most accurate way of reading agglutination tests when used by an experienced worker. The cell button is removed using a pipette and transferred to a microscope slide for examination. It is best to observe the cells using a relatively low power, such as a ×10 eyepiece with a ×10 objective, and observe moving fields. This may be achieved by gently tipping the slide or microscope so that the cells flow across the field of view. In inexperienced hands, the fragile red cell agglutinates can be easily disrupted by poor pipetting technique. Alternatively, the red cells can be gently resuspended using the tip and roll technique described above and then the contents of the tube tipped directly onto a microscope slide.

Reactions on slides. These require the direct mixing of red cells and serum on the slide. The tests require constant, gentle mixing by rotation of the slide, to allow maximum cell-to-cell contact for intercellular bridge formation. Slide tests are usually read macroscopically and are best used only for avid antibodies.

The use of microplates. This enables the dispensing of reagents and samples, and the reading of reactions, to be quite easily automated. Microplate tests use either liquid phase or solid phase techniques. Liquid phase tests are similar to tube tests except they are performed in the wells of the microplate. Solid phase tests require either red cells or antibody to be physically bound to the wells. As with tube tests, cells must be sedimented in the wells either by gravity or gentle centrifugation before being read macroscopically, by photometer or by an image analysis system.

Macroscopic examination. This may be achieved in several ways and may involve the use of an optical aid such as a magnifying mirror. The cells may be resuspended using gentle **agitation** of the microplate. This method is only advisable with the most avid antibodies such as monoclonal ABO and Rh typing sera. Another method is to observe the **settling pattern and streaming** of the red cells as the microplate is gently tipped. Irregular settling patterns with no streaming indicate a positive reaction, smooth settling patterns and streaming of cells on tipping indicate a negative reaction. A further method is to use a **photometer** to read the settling patterns using either single point, dual point or multipoint scanning of the microplate wells. Finally, an **image analysis** system, which records a 'picture' of each well and compares it with reference records of positive and negative settling patterns, may be used.

The use of microtubes

Several microtube systems (sometimes called card, cassette, column agglutination or gel tests) are available. All the systems consist of six narrow tubes each with a larger reaction chamber at the top, moulded into a plastic cassette or card. The tubes contain a density gradient material which allows red cells but not serum to pass through. In addition, the tubes contain either Sephadex gel or microbeads to trap agglutinated cells physically, or a substance such as protein G, which has a high affinity for IgG antibody, to trap IgG-coated red cells.

Cells and serum are incubated in the upper reaction chamber of the microtubes. After appropriate incubation, the cards are centrifuged and the

Table 10.2 An example of an agglutination scoring system for microtube tests

Score	Distribution of red cells in the microtube
4+	Layer of agglutinated cells on the top of the gel medium
3+	Agglutinated cells dispersed near the top of the gel medium
2+	Agglutinated cells dispersed through the entire length of the gel medium
1+	Agglutinated cells dispersed in the gel medium near the bottom of the column
0	A button of unagglutinated cells in the bottom of the tube

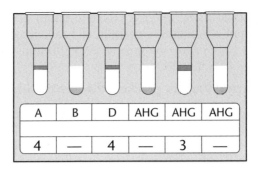

Figure 10.9
A microtube cassette showing positive (3+ and 4+) and negative (–) reactions.

red cells pass though the density gradient and into the trapping medium. Alternatively, typing sera may be incorporated into the microtubes so that red cells may be typed by immediate centrifugation into the matrix containing the antiserum, where they may be agglutinated and trapped. Also, AHG may be incorporated in the microtubes. As the density gradient only allows red cells to pass down the microtube, it is not necessary to wash the cells prior to contact with the AHG. Once again, the agglutinates or antibody-coated cells will be trapped whilst free cells pass through to form a layer at the bottom of the microtube. An example of an agglutination scoring system for microtubes is shown in *Table 10.2*.

Microtube tests may be examined macroscopically (see *Fig. 10.9*). Once the tubes have been centrifuged, the reactions are stable for many hours or even days and so may be read when convenient. The centrifuged cards may be kept for later inspection by another worker or a supervisor if the results require a second opinion. Alternatively, the reactions may be read by an image analysis system. At the time of writing, microtube methods are the most widely used method in the UK.

10.5 ASSOCIATED TECHNICAL CONSIDERATIONS

Enhancement of reactions

Every enhancement method for detecting antigen/antibody reactions (e.g. LIS solutions, polybrene, enzymes), every preservative and every additive has associated with it examples of false or unwanted positive, or false negative reactions. The unwanted positive reactions are usually due to clinically insignificant antibodies only detectable with a particular technique or in the presence of a particular preservative. Well-reported examples include clinically insignificant antibodies reacting only in LIS-AGTs, antibodies which react only in the presence of EDTA (or absence of calcium) and antibodies which react only in the presence of antibiotic preservatives such as chloramphenicol. No single antibody detection method will detect all red cell antibodies; for instance, MN and Duffy system antibodies cannot be detected using enzyme techniques and polybrene methods may miss Kell system antibodies. Generally, the more ingredients and variables there are in a test system, the greater is the likelihood of false results.

Serum versus plasma for antibody detection

Traditionally, serum has been used in blood group serology for the detection of red cell antibodies. Clotted samples are simple to collect and a possible variable, the anticoagulant, is avoided. The use of fully automated blood grouping systems has made it necessary to use anticoagulated samples, as the probes used to aspirate both plasma and cells cannot aspirate cells from clotted samples. Anticoagulated plasma has been shown to be acceptable for the detection of IgG antibodies. However, if the anticoagulant is a chelating agent such as ethylenediaminetetraacetic acid (EDTA) or citrate, then the detection of complement fixed by clinically significant antibodies is not possible. This is particularly a problem with clinically significant complement-fixing IgM antibodies, as they will not otherwise be detected in the AGT with modern polyspecific AHG (anti-IgG + anti-C3d). Additionally, antibody-mediated haemolysis of red cells in screening or compatibility testing usually indicates a potentially very dangerous red cell antibody. This haemolysis will not be detected if EDTA plasma is used. If the detection of clinically significant complement-fixing antibodies is considered to be desirable, then an anticoagulant which is less likely to interfere with complement fixing (e.g. heparin) may be used in place of EDTA or citrate.

Use of controls

Positive and negative controls are essential to show that test systems are working correctly. Controls should be processed under the same conditions as the tests. General guidance for the use of controls in blood group serology is given below.

When testing red cells for the presence of a particular blood group antigen using a typing serum, the following controls should be used: a **positive control** in which the typing serum is tested against red cells cell expressing a heterozygous or weak expression of the antigen being detected; and a **negative control** in which the typing serum is tested against red cells which are negative for the antigen being detected.

In addition, reactions with the patient's sample need to be controlled. When typing patient red cells, a negative control should be included of patient red cells reacted with patient's serum (auto-control) or reacted with an inert reagent control. This reagent control is essentially the inert diluent used for the typing serum. A positive reaction in this control (probably due to auto-agglutination or polyagglutination) invalidates any positive test results. When ABO grouping a patient, a negative control of the patient's serum with group O cells should be included. A positive result in this control indicates the presence of cold agglutinins other than anti-A or anti-B, and invalidates the test results. When performing crossmatching tests or antibody identifications, an auto-control of patient red cells with patient serum should be included. A negative result in this control indicates that any positive test result must be due to allo-antibody. A positive auto-control indicates that a positive test result may be due to an auto-antibody or auto-antibody + allo-antibody. In this case, further testing would be required to identify the problem.

Compatibility testing

This refers to all the procedures utilized in the selection and testing of a donor unit for transfusion to a patient. In this section, just those procedures relevant to this chapter will be highlighted.

ABO and Rh D typing. This test on both donor and patient is best performed using robust, direct agglutination techniques in normal saline. Usually monoclonal typing reagents are used in tubes, microplates or microtubes. Typically, equal volumes of serum/plasma and a 3% suspension of red cells in saline are used. The test may be performed manually or may be automated. Reading of results is usually macroscopic and may involve the use of photometers or image analysis systems.

Screening patient blood samples for clinically significant red cell antibodies. This is best performed using LIS-AGT or NIS-AGT at 37°C. The ratio of serum to cells should be at least 70:1. In the LIS-AGT, equal volumes of serum and cells must be used to maintain low ionic conditions. The tests are usually performed in microtubes or tubes, or in microplates using solid phase techniques. The tests may be performed manually or may be automated. Reading of microtube and microplate tests may be macroscopic or involve the use of photometers or image analysis systems. Reading of tube tests is usually microscopic. However, with less experienced workers, the tip and roll technique has been shown to give fewer false negative results than microscopic reading. This is because the removal and transfer of red cells from a tube to a microscope slide using a pipette can, in inexperienced hands, lead to disruption of agglutination.

Crossmatching. This involves testing patient serum/plasma against donor red cells and usually comprises a direct agglutination test and an AGT at 37°C. The direct agglutination test is performed immediately prior to incubating for the AGT. Its purpose is to rapidly indicate the presence of avid, direct agglutinating (complete) antibodies, especially those of the ABO system. The AGT, which may be LIS- or NIS-AGT, will detect clinically significant antibodies in most blood group systems (including ABO). Crossmatching tests are usually carried out in microtubes and either read macroscopically or with the aid of photometers or image analysis systems, or in tubes and read microscopically.

Antibody identification

A detailed review of the procedures for identifying blood group antibodies is beyond the scope of this introductory text. However, the principles outlined in this chapter should give the student sufficient background to appreciate the wide variety of techniques available, and their limitations, for the resolution of red cell antibodies.

SUGGESTED FURTHER READING

BCSH Blood Transfusion Task Force (2004) Guidelines for compatibility procedures in blood transfusion laboratories. *Transfusion Medicine* **14**, 59–73.

Knight, R.C. and De Silva, M. (1996) New technologies for red-cell serology. *Blood Reviews* **10**, 101–110.

Knight, R.C. and Poole, G.D. (1995) Detection of red cell antibodies: current and future techniques. *British Journal of Biomedical Science* **52**, 297–305.

van Oss, C.J. and Absolom, D.R. (1983) Zeta potentials, van der Waals forces and haemagglutination. *Vox Sanguinis* **44**, 183–190.

van Oss, V.J. (1994) Immunological and physiological nature of antigen-antibody interactions. In: *Immunobiology of Transfusion Medicine* (ed. G. Garratty). New York: Marcel Dekker.

Phillips, P.K., Voak, D., Whitton, C.M., Downie, D.M., Bebbington, C. and Campbell, J. (1993) BCSH-NIBSC anti-D reference reagent for antiglobulin tests: the in-house assessment of red cell washing centrifuges and of operator variability in the detection of weak, macroscopic agglutination. *Transfusion Medicine* **3**, 143–148.

SELF-ASSESSMENT QUESTIONS

1. Name three factors which affect the first stage of agglutination.
2. What are the most likely causes of a false negative antiglobulin test?
3. How does treatment of red cells with proteolytic enzymes help to bring about direct agglutination with IgG antibodies?
4. Name four of the bonds or forces involved in antibody binding.
5. Why are IgM antibodies generally more likely than IgG antibodies to bring about direct agglutination of red cells suspended in saline?

Adverse effects of blood transfusion

Learning objectives
After studying this chapter you should be able to:

■ Describe the importance of donor selection

■ List the tests performed on donor blood prior to release from the blood centre

■ List the tests performed at the hospital transfusion laboratory prior to transfusion

■ Describe the adverse effects due to red cell, platelet and plasma transfusions

■ Describe the laboratory investigation of an alleged red cell transfusion reaction

■ Outline the methods available to minimize the adverse effects of blood transfusion

The transfusion of the correct blood product, to the correct patient, at the correct time, can make an important contribution to a patient's well-being or recovery, and may even be life-saving. However, every transfusion carries a risk to the patient of adversely affecting the patient's well-being or recovery and may even be life-threatening.

When prescribing a blood transfusion or treatment with a product derived from human blood, the clinician must balance the potential benefits to the patient with the potential risks.

The responsibilities of the transfusion scientist in the transfusion process are evident at every stage in the chain from production to supply. They are intimately involved in the testing, treating, storing and issuing of blood products and in investigating adverse reactions. It is vitally important, therefore, that they appreciate and understand the risks of transfusion and how they may be eliminated or minimized.

This chapter will examine the general precautions which must be taken when selecting and testing donors, processing and storing blood products, performing pre-transfusion tests, monitoring transfusion episodes and reporting adverse events. It will also examine in more detail the adverse effects associated with the transfusion of red cells, leucocytes, platelets and plasma: disease transmission and other risks associated with blood transfusion. Ways of minimizing these risks are discussed and finally there is a section on the investigation of an alleged red cell transfusion reaction.

11.1 GENERAL PRECAUTIONS

The safety of all transfusions involves several elements. Those relating to the donor include the selection and testing of the donor; blood product collection or manufacture; blood product storage and transport; and pre-transfusion treatment of the blood product to reduce the risk of pathogen transmission, where appropriate. The elements relating to the patient are: the collection of the blood sample from the correct patient; pre-transfusion testing of the patient's sample; the selection of the appropriate blood product for the patient; accurately identifying the patient prior to transfusion; monitoring of the transfusion episode; and the reporting of any adverse events.

Donor selection

The process of donor selection is designed to protect both the donor and the recipient (see *Box 11.1*). In the UK, a donor must be a healthy person between the age of 17 and 70 years. They receive no payment for their donation. Donors either complete a questionnaire or are interviewed to identify those who could be harmed by donating and those whose donations could harm patients. The donor's haemoglobin (Hb) level is also checked. The acceptable lower limits for venous blood are 125 g l^{-1} for female donors and 135 g l^{-1} for male donors.

Box 11.1 Typical criteria used in the selection of donors

Donors are required to complete a questionnaire and answer a series of standard questions relating to their general health, lifestyle, past medical history and medication. Questions cover areas such as:

- lifestyle relating to high-risk sexual activity or drug taking
- recent body piercing/tattoos
- recent foreign travel
- previous blood transfusion (since 1980)
- family history of certain diseases
- current state of health/medications being taken

The emphasis is on identifying donors who carry a high risk for disease transmission, have a transmissible disorder, e.g. an allergy, or are taking medication which may affect the patient or the component being prepared. For example, the quality of platelet components will be adversely affected if the donor has been taking aspirin.

The system in the UK relies on the honesty of the donor, but as the intention of the overwhelming majority of donors is to help others, the system works well.

Since 1999, the UK blood service has sourced donor plasma for fractionated plasma products from areas of the world where there are few cases of bovine spongiform encephalopathy (BSE) and low risk of variant Creutzfeldt–Jakob disease (vCJD). In addition, this plasma is collected from areas whose donor populations have a low risk of viral disease. Currently, plasma used by UK manufacturers is sourced from the USA and Germany.

Donor testing

In the UK, all blood donations are subjected to mandatory tests for hepatitis B virus (HBV), hepatitis C virus (HCV), human immunodeficiency virus (HIV 1 and 2), human T cell leukemia virus (HTLV 1 and 2) and syphilis. Selected donations may also be tested for cytomegalovirus (CMV), for components to be transfused to neonates or immunocompromised patients (see *Box 11.2*). Blood donations are only released for issue to hospitals or fractionation centres for further processing if the results of these tests are negative.

Box 11.2 Disease-related tests performed on blood donors in the UK

Mandatory tests
- HBV by testing for HBsAg (surface antigen)
- HCV by testing for anti-HCV antibodies and HCV nucleic acid testing
- HIV 1 and 2 by testing for antibodies
- HTLV 1 and 2 by testing for antibodies
- Syphilis by *Treponema pallidum* haemagglutination assay (TPHA) testing for antibodies

Optional tests
- CMV by testing for antibodies
- Malaria by testing for antibodies
- *Trypanosoma cruzi* by testing for antibodies
- West Nile virus RNA

All transfusion centres in the UK conduct microbiological surveillance of the donation collection and processing procedures by taking appropriate samples for culture of microorganisms from the donor unit, the storage and the laboratory environment and equipment.

Blood donors have their ABO and Rh D types established at each donation. These results are compared with the results of previous tests (if any) held in a computer database. Blood is only released for issue if there is agreement between the current and historical results. The donor is also screened for atypical, clinically significant red cell antibodies. The blood is withheld if the results are positive.

Collection and storage

The blood donation must be collected as aseptically as possible, although total sterility is never achievable. The skin at the site of the venepuncture is cleansed with antiseptic, but bacteria below the surface of the skin may enter the venepuncture needle, as may airborne bacteria. It is also quite possible for the donor to have an asymptomatic bacteraemia at the time of donation and bacteria in the circulation of the donor will enter the donation. Some of these bacteria will be destroyed by the activity of leucocytes in the donation, and surviving bacteria will have their proliferation curtailed by storage at 4–6°C. There are, however, some bacteria which are capable of growth even at low temperatures, e.g. *Pseudomonas fluorescens* and *Yersinia enterocolitica*. The risk of bacterial proliferation increases if the blood bag is allowed to warm to ambient temperature. For this reason, transfusion must commence within 30 minutes of removal of the blood pack from the refrigerator, and be completed within 4 hours (for red cells). In addition, if the blood pack is removed from the refrigerator for further testing, processing or transportation, it must be returned to the correct storage temperature within 30 minutes to minimize the chance of bacterial proliferation within the pack. If the pack is allowed to warm for sufficient time for the bacteria to enter a logarithmic growth phase, then the bacterial load may have been increased by a factor of hundreds if not thousands. This situation will be exacerbated every time the blood pack is allowed to warm. Bacterial proliferation is an even greater problem with platelet components as these are stored at 22–24°C.

Bacteria may also enter components and plasma fractions during processing; for this reason, aseptic technique is again vital when handling and processing blood donations. At the blood transfusion centres, processing usually takes place in specially designed donation packs with hermetically sealed transfer bags for separation of the various components, or by the attachment of transfer bags using sterile docking procedures.

At the hospital transfusion laboratory, donor blood bags may have to be opened to allow removal of plasma or buffy coat, or to attach a leucocyte depletion filter. Again aseptic technique must be observed. Correct storage conditions after opening are essential to reduce the risk of bacterial proliferation, as are strict controls on the maximum time of storage following the opening of a blood bag. These times are usually 12 hours for red cells when stored between 4°C and 6°C after opening and 6 hours for platelets stored between 22°C and 24°C.

At the patient's bedside, the blood bags are opened to allow attachment of the blood-giving set. Aseptic technique is essential during this process.

Blood product selection, pre-treatment and pre-transfusion testing

The patient should be transfused with the most appropriate therapeutic product for their clinical condition. A wide range of blood products is available and it is important to be aware of the most appropriate product, its availability and the current guidelines for use. (See Chapter 9 for more detailed information on the selection of appropriate therapeutic product.)

Pre-transfusion testing of the patient usually takes place at the hospital transfusion laboratory. The patient's ABO and Rh D type are established and the patient's serum or plasma sample is screened for atypical, clinically significant red cell antibodies.

In the case of red cell transfusions, the patient's serum or plasma is tested against the donor red cells (crossmatched) by techniques designed to detect incompatibility due to ABO or other clinically significant red cell antibodies. Blood is usually only released for transfusion if these tests are negative.

Clerical errors may occur when taking the pre-transfusion blood sample from the patient, during laboratory testing or when transfusing blood. These errors are the most common causes of incompatible transfusions. The UK Serious Hazards of Transfusion (SHOT) report from 2005 indicates that approximately 42% of near-miss events were due to misidentification of the patient when collecting the blood sample. Analysis of incidents in which the incorrect blood component was transfused showed that 18% were due to blood being transfused to the wrong patient and in 57% of these cases, the pre-transfusion checks had not been performed correctly. Analysis of laboratory testing errors showed that 44% were due to the selection of the wrong patient sample.

Monitoring of transfusions and reporting of adverse incidents

Patients receiving a transfusion of any blood product must be monitored closely for the first 15 minutes of each unit transfused. In this way, early clinical signs of acute reactions to incompatibilities or bacterial contamination can be detected. The patient's temperature, pulse, blood pressure and respiration should be recorded before and after each transfusion episode and after the first 15 minutes of each unit transfused. The patient should continue to be monitored regularly during and after the transfusion, to detect any signs of delayed reactions.

All used transfusion bags should be retained for a minimum of 24 hours after the blood transfusion is completed so that they are available for re-testing in the event of any adverse reaction to the transfusion. If an adverse reaction is suspected during or after a transfusion, the hospital transfusion laboratory should be informed as soon as possible so that appropriate investigations can be instigated without delay (see *Box 11.3*; see also *Box 11.5* concerning pre-treatment of blood products to minimize adverse reactions).

Suspected bacterial or viral infections caused by transfusion are reported as a matter of urgency to the local blood transfusion centre. In addition, these and other serious adverse reactions such as acute or delayed haemolysis, and anaphylactic reactions, which result from the transfusion of blood components (see *Box 11.5*), should be reported to both the Medicines and Healthcare products Regulatory Agency (MHRA) using the

---

Box 11.3 Definitions of adverse reactions and events as reportable to the MHRA in the UK

Serious adverse reactions are unintended responses in a donor or patient which are associated with the collection or transfusion of blood or blood components. The reaction may be fatal, life-threatening, disabling or incapacitating, or result in or prolong hospitalization or morbidity.

Serious adverse events are any untoward occurrences associated with the collection, testing, processing, storage and distribution of blood or blood components that might lead to death or life-threatening, disabling or incapacitating conditions for patients, or which might result in or prolong hospitalization or morbidity.

Examples are:

- haemolysis due to blood group antibodies
- other causes of haemolysis
- transfusion-transmitted bacterial, viral or parasitic infection
- anaphylaxis or hypersensitivity
- transfusion-related acute lung injury (TRALI)
- post-transfusion purpura
- graft-versus-host disease (GVHD)
- other serious reaction(s) such as circulatory overload

Serious Adverse Blood Reactions and Events (SABRE) system and the SHOT group. SHOT is a voluntary, anonymized system which aims to collect data on serious adverse events of transfusion of blood components, and to make recommendations to improve transfusion safety, using their confidential reporting system. The MHRA is the UK Competent Authority for Blood Safety as defined by the EU Blood Safety Directive.

11.2 ADVERSE EFFECTS CAUSED BY TRANSMISSION OF INFECTIOUS AGENTS

The transfusion of blood products carries the risk of transmitting viral, bacterial or protozoal infections from the donor to the patient.

Viral infections. Those most often reported in association with blood transfusion include HIV, HBV, HCV, CMV, hepatitis A virus (HAV), Epstein–Barr virus (EBV) and parvovirus B19. Testing donors for HIV, HTLV, HBV and HCV is mandatory but donors in the 'window period' of an infection may not be detected. The 'window period' is that time between infection and the development of detectable specific antibodies when a donor is infectious but is still negative with respect to a particular virus.

The risks may be minimized by the careful selection of donors, laboratory testing for HIV, HTLV, HBV, HCV and CMV, and pathogen reduction methods such as heat and/or chemical treatment and solvent/detergent treatment of plasma fractions to inactivate enveloped viruses. Leucocyte depletion of red cell and platelet components will reduce the risk of CMV transmission as the virus is carried within leucocytes. The risk of transmitting HAV and parvovirus B19 is reduced in plasma pools as up to 60% of normal donors have antibodies to these viruses in their plasma.

Bacterial infections. Those transmitted by blood transfusion can rapidly be fatal for the patient. As previously mentioned, bacteria may enter the blood supply at the time of collection or during subsequent processing. Some bacteria, e.g. *Yersinia enterocolitica*, are capable of proliferating even during storage of blood at 4°C.

The risks may be minimized by careful selection of donors, laboratory testing in the case of *Treponema pallidum*, the causative agent for syphilis, and microbiological surveillance of the donor, storage and testing environments. Strict adherence to storage temperatures, not allowing blood to be out of refrigerated storage conditions for more than 30 minutes prior to transfusion, limiting storage times after components have been opened for processing, and adopting aseptic techniques during processing all contribute to minimizing the risk of bacterial infection.

Protozoal infections. Those most often reported in connection with blood transfusion include malaria, babeiosis, toxoplasmosis and filariasis. No laboratory testing procedures for these organisms are routinely conducted in the UK. The risks of transmission are minimised by careful donor selection and the rejection of donors who have recently visited areas where any of these infections are endemic.

11.3 ADVERSE REACTIONS DUE TO THE TRANSFUSION OF RED CELLS

The most serious reaction to a red cell transfusion (see *Fig. 11.1*) is that of **acute intravascular haemolysis** of the donor red cells by haemolytic anti-red cell antibodies in the patient. These are usually ABO system antibodies. The destruction of red cells, activation of complement and release of haemoglobin leads rapidly to disseminated intravascular coagulation, acute renal failure and shock, and is fatal in at least 10% of cases. The majority of ABO-incompatible transfusions occur due to clerical errors in the identification of the patient at the time of sampling, collection of blood from the laboratory or at the time of transfusion.

The risk may be minimized by ensuring:

- accurate blood grouping and labelling of donor units
- accurate blood grouping of patients
- pre-transfusion testing to detect ABO or other haemolytic antibodies
- accurate identification of the patient at the time of sampling
- accurate identification of the patient and donor unit at the time of collection from the laboratory
- accurate identification of the patient prior to transfusion

Delayed (extravascular) haemolysis. This reaction to transfused red cells may be caused by antibodies to several different blood group systems (see Chapter 6). The patient's haemoglobin level will fall as the transfused donor red cells are destroyed and the patient may suffer from a fever and general malaise. Future transfusions require red cells which have been typed for

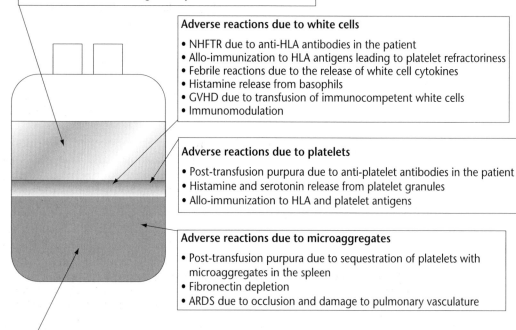

Adverse reactions due to plasma

• Anaphylactic shock due to anti-IgA antibody in the patient
• Allergic reactions due to the transfusion of allergens
• Febrile reactions due to cytokines from effete white cells
• TRALI due to donor anti-granulocyte antibodies

Adverse reactions due to white cells

• NHFTR due to anti-HLA antibodies in the patient
• Allo-immunization to HLA antigens leading to platelet refractoriness
• Febrile reactions due to the release of white cell cytokines
• Histamine release from basophils
• GVHD due to transfusion of immunocompetent white cells
• Immunomodulation

Adverse reactions due to platelets

• Post-transfusion purpura due to anti-platelet antibodies in the patient
• Histamine and serotonin release from platelet granules
• Allo-immunization to HLA and platelet antigens

Adverse reactions due to microaggregates

• Post-transfusion purpura due to sequestration of platelets with microaggregates in the spleen
• Fibronectin depletion
• ARDS due to occlusion and damage to pulmonary vasculature

Adverse reactions due to red cells

• Acute intravascular haemolysis due to ABO antibodies
• Extravascular haemolysis and delayed reactions due to other red cell antibodies
• Allo-immunization to red cell antigens
• Iron overload

Figure 11.1
Adverse reaction risks with the transfusion of red cell products (see text for full details).

blood group antigens and shown to be negative with respect to the patient's antibody.

The risk may be minimized by performing pre-transfusion screening of the patient's serum/plasma for clinically significant red cell antibodies and crossmatching the patient's serum/plasma against the donor red cells.

Allo-immunization. This reaction to many different red cell antigens will occur at every transfusion as the donor red cells will normally only be matched with the patient's ABO and Rh D type. After a patient has received a transfusion of red cells, any further transfusions should be preceded by antibody screening and crossmatching with a sample taken at least 3 days after the last transfusion. This is to allow sufficient time for any newly formed antibodies to appear in the serum/plasma. If a patient does develop red cell antibodies this could lead to difficulties in supplying blood in the future or to haemolytic disease of the newborn in subsequent pregnancies.

The risk may be minimized by only transfusing red cells when absolutely necessary, treating the patient with iron rather than red cells to correct iron deficiency anaemia, or the use of recombinant erythropoietin, a growth factor which stimulates the patient's own red cell production.

Iron overload. This is a particular risk for patients who receive regular red cell transfusions over many months or years. The accumulation of iron from transfused red cells can lead to widespread tissue damage and interference with hepatic function. The risk may be minimized by treating the patient with chelation therapy using, for example, desferrioxamine, to eliminate unwanted iron.

Box 11.4 Delayed transfusion reaction

An 85-year-old female (CG) was admitted to hospital on 26 February for elective total hip replacement surgery. On admission, she had a low haemoglobin (Hb) level of 85 g l⁻¹ and a raised mean cell volume (MCV) of 105 fl. A blood film examination indicated a possible folate deficiency. She was immediately started on folate and vitamin B12 treatment and transfused with two units of red cells. Surgery was deferred.

At this time, CG grouped as O Rh D positive with no clinically significant antibodies detected. The two units of red cells were compatible in the crossmatch and were transfused uneventfully.

On 14 May, the patient was re-admitted. Her Hb was now 120 g l⁻¹ with an MCV of 103 fl. No clinically significant antibodies were detected in her serum and two units of crossmatch-compatible red cells were transfused uneventfully during surgery on 18 May.

Post-operatively on 21 May, her Hb had fallen to 88 g l⁻¹, although there had been no significant post-operative blood loss. She complained of feeling generally unwell and had a slight fever, although there was no evidence of a post-operative infection. A sample was sent for crossmatching of red cells to correct the anaemia. The units of red cells crossmatched were found to be incompatible (that is, positive results were detected) in the indirect antiglobulin test and the auto-control (a test of patient's red cells with patient's own serum) was positive.

On further investigation, the patient's serum was shown to contain the Rh antibody anti-E. The direct antiglobulin test (DAT) performed on the patient's red cell sample was positive with an IgG antibody shown to be coating the red cells. This antibody was eluted from the red cells and was identified as anti-E.

Two units of O Rh D-positive, E-negative red cells were crossmatched and found to be compatible. CG was transfused with both units uneventfully on 27 May. Her Hb rose to 122 g l⁻¹ and remained steady throughout the rest of her hospital stay.

Explanation

The patient had been immunized by the transfusion of E-positive red cells to correct the pre-operative anaemia on 4 March. The anti-E produced as a result of this immunization was too weak to be detected when red cells were crossmatched for the surgery on 18 May. One or both of the units transfused during surgery on 18 May were positive for the E antigen. The patient did not react immediately to this fresh immunization but had a delayed reaction caused by a secondary antibody response, 3 days later, which caused a fall in her Hb level as the transfused red cells were destroyed by her antibody. The positive DAT was detecting the patient's antibody bound to transfused donor red cells still in her circulation. The transfusion of red cells which were negative with respect to her anti-E antibody successfully corrected her anaemia.

11.4 ADVERSE REACTIONS DUE TO THE TRANSFUSION OF LEUCOCYTES

There are several different types of adverse reaction which can occur following transfusion of blood containing leucocytes. These include non-haemolytic febrile transfusion reactions, post-transfusion purpura, acute respiratory distress syndrome, graft-versus-host disease, allo-immunization and immunomodulation.

Non-haemolytic febrile transfusion reactions (NHFTR). Prior to universal leucodepletion of donated blood, NHFTR used to occur in the UK in as many as 1% of all transfusions and in up to 45% of patients receiving multiple transfusions. Patients may experience flushing, pyrexia, rigors and hypotension. The reactions are caused by anti-leucocyte antibodies in the patient reacting with donor leucocytes to activate complement causing the release of pyrogens and vasoactive amines. Similar reactions can occur due to the **release of cytokines** from damaged donor leucocytes. Likewise, **histamine** released from effete donor basophils may cause urticarial reactions or bronchospasm and hypotension in the patient. These risks may be minimized by removing the donor leucocytes (leucodepletion) from any red cell or platelet components prior to transfusion.

Post-transfusion purpura (PTP). PTP may occur due to the sequestration of platelets into the spleen in association with transfused microaggregates. These microaggregates occur in all donations of red cells and comprise an aggregate of fibrin, donor leucocytes and platelets. The number and size of these aggregates increases with the length of storage of the donated blood. Microaggregates have also been implicated in **reducing fibronectin levels** in transfused patients. The risk may be minimized by removal of microaggregates by filtration immediately prior to transfusion, particularly for patients receiving massive transfusions.

Adult respiratory distress syndrome (ARDS). ARDS may be caused by occlusion of the pulmonary vasculature by transfused microaggregates. This can lead to the release of free oxygen radicals, release of lysosomal enzymes and complement activation with consequent damage to the lungs. The risk may be minimized by removal of microaggregates by filtration immediately prior to transfusion, particularly in patients receiving massive transfusions.

Graft-versus-host disease (GVHD). GVHD is an often fatal condition brought about by the transfusion of immunocompetent leucocytes to an immunocompromised patient. The donor leucocytes (the graft) proliferate in the patient (the host) and reject a variety of host tissues (see Chapter 12). The risk may be minimized by irradiating red cell and platelet components prior to transfusion to kill the donor leucocytes.

Allo-immunization. Allo-immunization to many different leucocyte antigens will occur at every transfusion of cellular blood components. This may lead to the production of antibodies to HLA (see Chapter 12), which are not only implicated in the NHFTR mentioned previously, but which may also cause the patient to become **refractory to platelet transfusions**. That is to say, the anti-HLA antibodies can destroy transfused platelets so that the patient does not get the expected benefit from the transfusions. In this case, the patient would have to be transfused with platelets from an HLA-matched donor. Finding suitable HLA-matched donors can be very difficult, time-consuming and expensive. The risk of allo-immunization may be minimized by removing the donor leucocytes (leucodepletion) from any red cell or platelet components prior to transfusion. This is especially important for patients who are receiving long-term red cell or platelet transfusion support.

Immunomodulation. Immunomodulation following transfusion refers to a temporary impairment of the patient's immune system. This may manifest itself in the form of an increased chance of tumour recurrence following surgery for tumour removal, or an increased incidence of post-operative infections, in patients receiving blood transfusions. The precise mechanism of this effect is unknown, but the most popular theories attribute the effect to the transfusion of leucocytes. The risk may be minimized by removing the donor leucocytes from any red cell or platelet components prior to transfusion.

11.5 ADVERSE REACTIONS DUE TO THE TRANSFUSION OF PLATELETS

These can occur for a variety of reasons (see *Fig. 11.2*).

Allo-immunization. Allo-immunization to many different platelet antigens will occur at every transfusion. This may lead to the production of anti-platelet antibodies. Platelet components may be contaminated with red cells and leucocytes, which may stimulate the patient to produce anti-red cell or anti-HLA antibodies. The anti-HLA antibodies may cause the patient to become refractory to platelet transfusions as described in Section 11.4.

The risk may be minimized by:

* selecting platelets from Rh D-negative donors for transfusion to Rh D females of childbearing age, to prevent the patient being immunized to produce anti-D
* the administration of prophylactic anti-D to any Rh D-negative female of childbearing age who has received platelets from an Rh D-positive donor
* removing the donor leucocytes from platelet components prior to transfusion to avoid the patient being stimulated to produce antibodies to HLA

Post-transfusion purpura (PTP). PTP is caused by platelet antibodies present in the patient and may result in a life-threatening thrombocytopenia. The risk may be minimized by the selection of platelets from matched donors once the anti-platelet antibody has been identified.

Histamine and serotonin release. Histamine and serotonin from damaged donor platelets can cause urticaria, bronchospasm and hypotension. There

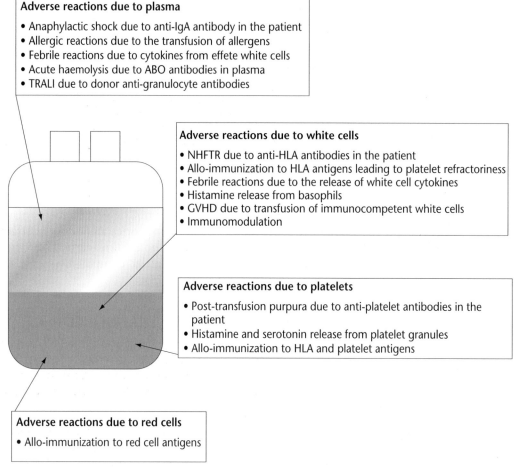

Adverse reactions due to plasma

- Anaphylactic shock due to anti-IgA antibody in the patient
- Allergic reactions due to the transfusion of allergens
- Febrile reactions due to cytokines from effete white cells
- Acute haemolysis due to ABO antibodies in plasma
- TRALI due to donor anti-granulocyte antibodies

Adverse reactions due to white cells

- NHFTR due to anti-HLA antibodies in the patient
- Allo-immunization to HLA antigens leading to platelet refractoriness
- Febrile reactions due to the release of white cell cytokines
- Histamine release from basophils
- GVHD due to transfusion of immunocompetent white cells
- Immunomodulation

Adverse reactions due to platelets

- Post-transfusion purpura due to anti-platelet antibodies in the patient
- Histamine and serotonin release from platelet granules
- Allo-immunization to HLA and platelet antigens

Adverse reactions due to red cells

- Allo-immunization to red cell antigens

Figure 11.2
Adverse reaction risks with the transfusion of platelet products (see text for details).

is no specific measure available to minimize this risk, but fortunately the symptoms are usually not severe and may be treated with anti-histamines.

Acute haemolysis. Destruction of patient red cells by donor ABO antibodies present in the supernatant plasma of the platelet component is a potential hazard but fortunately this is a rare occurrence. The risk may be minimized by selecting platelets from ABO-compatible donors.

11.6   ADVERSE REACTIONS DUE TO THE TRANSFUSION OF PLASMA

These can also occur for a variety of reasons (see *Fig 11.3*).

Anaphylactic shock reactions. These extreme allergic reactions are rare but have a high mortality rate. They are usually caused by a reaction between

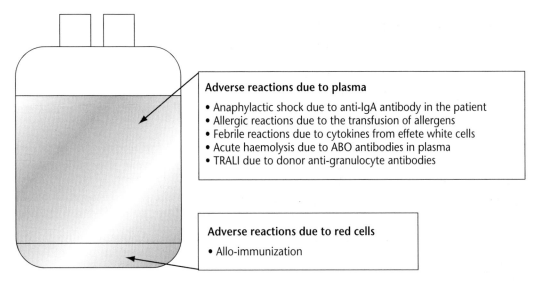

Adverse reactions due to plasma

- Anaphylactic shock due to anti-IgA antibody in the patient
- Allergic reactions due to the transfusion of allergens
- Febrile reactions due to cytokines from effete white cells
- Acute haemolysis due to ABO antibodies in plasma
- TRALI due to donor anti-granulocyte antibodies

Adverse reactions due to red cells

- Allo-immunization

Figure 11.3
Adverse reaction risks with the transfusion of plasma products (see text for details).

IgE anti-IgA in the patient's serum, particularly if they are IgA-deficient, and the IgA contained in the transfused plasma. The risk may be minimized by using products from IgA-deficient donors for future transfusions and/or by transfusing red cells and platelet components which have been washed free of plasma.

Transfusion-related acute lung injury (TRALI). This is most usually caused by antibodies to polymorphonuclear leucocytes (PMN) in the donor plasma reacting with the patient's PMN. Complement is activated and PMN breakdown occurs primarily in the pulmonary vasculature leading to non-cardiogenic pulmonary oedema and infiltration of the lower lung. The condition is potentially fatal.

The risk may be minimized by:

- identifying donors who have been implicated in cases of TRALI and removing them from the regular donor panels
- sourcing of fresh frozen plasma (FFP) from untransfused male donors (as they will not have developed anti-granulocyte antibodies)
- suspending platelets in a plasma-free medium
- reducing inappropriate use of FFP by closely following transfusion guidelines

Mild allergic reactions. These reactions to plasma, whether from FFP, platelet or red cell supernatant, are very common and are usually either caused by the reaction between an allergen in the transfused plasma and patient antibody or, more rarely, by an allergy passively acquired from the donor. The risk may be minimized by careful selection of donors to eliminate those with known allergies.

Febrile reactions. These may also occur due to the presence of cytokines which have been released into the plasma from damaged donor leucocytes. The risk may be minimized by removing the donor leucocytes from any red cell or platelet components (preferably pre-storage).

Allo-immunization to red cell antigens. This may occur due to the small amounts of red cell stroma found in some FFP preparations. The risks may be minimized by:

- selecting FFP from Rh D-negative donors for transfusion to Rh D-negative females of childbearing age, to prevent the patient being immunized to produce anti-D
- the administration of prophylactic anti-D to any Rh D-negative female of childbearing age who has received FFP from an Rh D-positive donor

Acute haemolysis of patient red cells by donor ABO antibodies present in FFP may also occur. The risk may be minimized by selection of FFP from ABO-compatible donors.

11.7 ADVERSE REACTIONS DUE TO OTHER CAUSES

Circulatory overload, **air embolism** and **thrombophlebitis** at the infusion site are conditions which may complicate all intravenous infusions. The risk is minimized by good clinical practice.

Toxicity caused by the transfusion of citrate in the anticoagulant or potassium which has leaked from red cells may be a problem for patients receiving massive transfusions in a short space of time. Toxicity caused by PVC or phthalate plasticizers which dissolve from the blood pack into the donor blood are a theoretical rather than a practical risk with modern blood packs.

Unusual reactions include reports of patients who developed **acute hypersensitivity reactions** during transfusion. These reactions were due to the patients having an IgE antibody which acted against residual ethylene oxide contained in the blood-giving sets. The ethylene oxide had been used to sterilize the giving sets. Patients have also been reported who developed an **urticarial rash** due to sensitivity to the nickel coating on the transfusion needle.

A much more serious risk is that of **hypothermia** and **cardiac arrest** brought on by the rapid transfusion of large volumes of cold blood. This risk may be minimized by the use of a blood warmer at the time of transfusion.

11.8 INVESTIGATION OF AN ALLEGED REACTION TO A RED CELL TRANSFUSION

The most common adverse reactions are not due to red cell antibodies but are febrile or urticarial reactions due to anti-leucocyte antibodies, cytokines or allergens.

Box 11.5 Pre-treatment of blood products to minimize the risks of an adverse reaction

Leucocyte depletion

Removal of leucocytes from red cell and platelet components prior to transfusion has been standard practice in the UK since 1999. It reduces the risk of an adverse reaction in several ways.

Pre-storage leucocyte depletion (the system adopted in the UK for universal leucodepletion) refers to the removal of leucocytes from the donation, usually by filtration, 24 to 72 hours **after collection**. This process can reduce the risk of:

- immunization to HLA antigens carried on the leucocytes
- febrile reactions caused by a patient's anti-HLA antibodies reacting with donor leucocytes
- CMV transmission, as the virus is carried in leucocytes
- impairment of the patient's immune system (immunomodulation)
- febrile reactions caused by cytokines released into the donor plasma from effete donor leucocytes
- reactions caused by the release of histamine into the donor plasma from effete donor basophils
- prion transmission, e.g. vCJD, theoretically at least

Post-storage leucocyte depletion refers to the removal of leucocytes from red cell or platelet components, usually by filtration, immediately **prior to transfusion**, either in the laboratory or at the bedside. This process can reduce the risk of:

- immunization to HLA antigens carried on the leucocytes
- febrile reactions caused by a patient's anti-HLA antibodies reacting with donor leucocytes
- CMV transmission, as the virus is carried in leucocytes
- impairment of the patient's immune system (immunomodulation)

The 1993 consensus conference of the Royal College of Physicians of Edinburgh recommended a level of less than 5×10^6 residual leucocytes per red cell unit or platelet dose for effective leucocyte depletion in most cases. Modern leucocyte depletion filters are capable of achieving this level by removing more than 99.9% of leucocytes from a blood donation.

Irradiation

Treating red cell or platelet components with gamma radiation removes the risk of GvHD by inactivating immunocompetent donor leucocytes. The British Committee for Standards in Haematology (1996) recommends that each component bag should receive a dose of gamma radiation of not less than 25 Gy and not more than 50 Gy.

Pathogen reduction

Reducing pathogens in donor plasma to lower the risk of disease transmission may be achieved in several ways. For example, plasma fractions and plasma pools may be treated with heat or with a combination of solvent and detergent. Fresh frozen plasma may be treated with methylene blue which irreversibly denatures viral DNA and RNA on exposure to white light. Research is ongoing into inactivation techniques for cellular and plasma products based on compounds such as psoralen and riboflavin that penetrate the genetic material (DNA or RNA) of microorganisms, including viruses, and then bind inextricably with it. As a result, the microorganisms are no longer able to proliferate.

These types of reaction also account for most of the immediate (or during transfusion) reactions and are usually not life-threatening, although they may be very uncomfortable and disconcerting for the patient. Immediate reactions caused by bacterial contamination or red cell incompatibility (usually ABO) are much rarer occurrences but can be rapidly fatal.

A more common occurrence when red cell antibodies are present is the delayed transfusion reaction, which may become apparent 3–14 days post-transfusion. It may only be detected because of a falling haemoglobin level due to destruction of transfused red cells, spherocytes in a blood smear, or a positive DAT or positive auto-control in a subsequent crossmatch (see Chapter 9). A delayed transfusion reaction is caused by a delayed secondary antibody response in the patient to the transfused red cells. Pre-transfusion, the antibody is at such a low level as to be not detectable.

Reactions which occur during a transfusion should be reported to the hospital transfusion laboratory, preferably as soon as possible after they occur and after the patient has been stabilized. The transfusion laboratory must then obtain a relevant history from the patient. This should include information concerning any previous transfusions, previous reactions, any history of haemolytic disease of the newborn, previous pregnancies, drugs and medication currently being taken.

In addition, they should obtain from the patient pre- and post-transfusion serum/plasma samples, a post-transfusion DAT sample and a post-transfusion urine sample. The laboratory should also obtain the remains of any used blood packs and the remains of the offending unit of blood with the blood-giving set still *in situ*. The blood in the pack will be examined for bacterial contamination. Leaving the giving set still attached to the blood

Table 11.1 Tests required for the investigation of an alleged reaction to a red cell transfusion

Sample	Tests
Pre-transfusion blood sample from the patient	• Repeat ABO and Rh group • Repeat antibody screen • Identify any antibodies detected • Repeat crossmatch of all units of blood
Post-transfusion blood sample from the patient	• ABO and Rh group • Antibody screen • Identify any antibodies detected • DAT • Crossmatch of all units of blood
Donor blood units	• Check for correct labelling of units of blood • Check ABO and Rh group • Antigen type for any antibodies found in pre- or post-transfusion samples
Post-transfusion urine sample from the patient	• Examine for signs of haemolysis
The offending unit of blood	• Send for microbiological testing (this usually involves testing samples from the pack, side tube and giving set)

Table 11.2 Tests required for the investigation of an alleged reaction to a red cell transfusion, when only the post-transfusion sample is available

Sample	Tests
Post-transfusion blood sample from the patient	• ABO and Rh group • Antibody screen • DAT • Identify any antibodies found • Blood smear to check for spherocytes

pack prevents any new bacterial contamination of the blood. Finally, any untransfused units of blood should be recovered and tests performed as shown in *Table 11.1*.

Sometimes, the pre-transfusion samples and donor units may no longer be available. In this case, the post-transfusion samples should be tested as shown in *Table 11.2*. Further more elaborate tests may need to be performed in addition to the tests shown in these tables, but these are beyond the scope of this introductory text.

11.9 SUMMARY

After reading this chapter, students may be forgiven for wondering how any patient ever survives a blood transfusion. The dangers and complications of transfusion are myriad, but in practice the vast majority of transfusions are uneventful. This is due to the knowledge and skills of the staff of the blood transfusion centres, fractionation centres and hospital blood transfusion laboratories, and of course to the commitment and honesty of the blood donors.

Techniques available to detect clinically significant antibodies, to prepare safe and effective blood products, to minimize disease transmission and reduce the other risks associated with blood transfusion are now very sophisticated. However, the transfusion community must not become complacent. There are still risks which need to be investigated and minimized, such as immunomodulation and the risk of virus transmission in red cell and platelet components. Adverse reactions are under-reported by nursing and clinical staff, so the real frequency of occurrence of many types of adverse reaction is still unknown.

SUGGESTED FURTHER READING

James, V. (ed.) (2005) *Guidelines for the Blood Transfusion Services in the United Kingdom*, 7th edn. London: TSO.

McClelland, D.B.L. (ed.) (2007) *Handbook of Transfusion Medicine*, 4th edn. London: United Kingdom Blood Services/TSO.

Medicines and Healthcare products Regulatory Agency: www.mhra.gov.uk
National Blood Service (UK): http://www.blood.co.uk
Serious Hazards of Transfusion Annual Report 2005. Published 30th November
    2006; ISBN 0 9532 789 8 0
Serious Hazards of Transfusion: http://www.shotuk.org
The British Committee for Standards in Haematology:
    http://www.bcshguidelines.com
UK Blood Transfusion and Tissue Transplantation Services; Professional
    Guidelines: http://www.transfusionguidelines.org.uk

SELF-ASSESSMENT QUESTIONS

1. In the UK, which mandatory disease-related tests are performed on all blood donations?
2. What is the most common cause of an incompatible red cell transfusion?
3. To whom should adverse transfusion reaction be reported?
4. How could the risk of GVHD be minimized?
5. Apart from allo-immunization and reactions to red cell antibodies, what is the other major danger of repeated red cell transfusions?
6. Describe the two mechanisms by which post-transfusion purpura may occur in a patient?
7. How may the risk of viral transmission from transfusion be minimized?
8. Describe which tests should be performed on the patient's post-transfusion samples following an alleged red cell transfusion reaction.
9. Briefly discuss the advantage of leucodepleting blood on the day after collection rather than immediately before transfusion.

12

Haemopoietic stem cell processing and transplantation

Learning objectives
After studying this chapter you should be able to:

■ Define what is meant by a haemopoietic stem cell transplant

■ Outline the reasons for carrying out a haemopoietic stem cell transplant

■ Discuss the different sources of haemopoietic stem cells for transplantation

■ Outline methods for obtaining and processing haemopoietic stem cells for transplantation

■ Discuss problems associated with haemopoietic stem cell transplantation

■ Discuss mechanisms for the prevention and treatment of graft-versus-host disease.

■ Describe the HLA system and discuss its polymorphic nature

■ Outline methods for tissue typing

12.1 INTRODUCTION

Haemopoietic stem cells (HSC) are those cells that are the progenitors of the cellular components in the blood, i.e. the red cells, the leucocytes and the platelets. Under the control of cytokines, these cells are constantly dividing and their progeny developing into different blood components. Those stem cells whose progeny can give rise to any of the blood cells are said to be **pluripotent**. They give rise to further stem cells whose progeny are more restricted in their development.

Transplants of tissues from one human to another have been carried out with a degree of success since Joseph Murray performed the first successful kidney transplant in 1954 (see *Table 12.1*). Nowadays, kidney and heart transplants have become more frequent and the range of tissues transplanted is extensive (see *Table 12.2*). Although tissue transplants are becoming routine, the process is not without its difficulties, the most obvious one being that if the graft comes from an individual who is not genetically identical to the recipient (as, for example, when a graft is carried out

Table 12.1 Some landmarks in clinical transplantation

Year	Landmark
1943	Medawar establishes that the immune system causes graft rejection
1954	First successful human kidney transplant
1958	Discovery of HLA antigens
1967	First human heart transplant
1968	First successful human bone marrow transplant from related donor
1968	First human liver transplants
1973	First successful bone marrow transplant from unrelated donor
1977	Use of autologous bone marrow reported
1986	First peripheral blood stem cell transplant
1987	First umbilical cord stem cell transplant
1990	E. Donnall Thomas wins Nobel prize for medicine for treatment of aplastic anaemia with bone marrow transplants

Table 12.2 Tissue and organ transplants

Tissue transplanted	Examples of clinical condition
Skin	Plastic surgery, e.g. for treatment of burns
Cornea	Types of blindness
Kidney	End-stage renal failure
Heart	Coronary heart disease
Heart and lungs	Cystic fibrosis
Pancreas	Insulin-dependent diabetes mellitus
Liver	Cirrhosis
Bone marrow and haemopoietic stem cells	Immune deficiency; leukaemia; myelodysplasia; aplastic anaemia
Bone	Orthopaedic surgery
Foetal brain cell	Parkinson's disease*
Foetal thymus	Immune deficiency*

*Experimental.

between identical twins, a rare event), then the immune system of the recipient is highly likely to destroy the transplanted tissues, which are recognized as foreign or 'non-self'.

The most common types of graft, which include kidney, heart, liver, lungs, pancreas and corneal transplants, are those in which the aim is to replace a defective organ. Such grafts are invariably given to people who have a properly functioning immune system. In these cases, the person who receives the graft is likely to mount an immune response against the graft, unless the graft is antigenically identical to the tissues of the donor or, if not, immunosuppressive treatments are given. Transplants of haemopoietic tissues, first successfully undertaken in 1968, present particular problems if the donor and recipient are not matched very closely. These problems arise because haemopoietic tissue contains small lymphocytes, or can give rise to small lymphocytes, which can recognize antigens on the host as foreign and mount an attack on the cells of the recipient. Such an occurrence is called a **graft-versus-host reaction** and it results in **graft-versus-host disease (GVHD)**, which can be fatal.

This chapter will look at the clinical circumstances in which haemopoietic stem cell transplants may be undertaken, the sources of such tissues and the ways in which the stem cells are identified and processed in the laboratory. In addition, this chapter will examine the immunological basis of graft rejection and how this relates to haemopoietic stem cell transplantation and will address the ways in which GVHD can be prevented and/or treated. This will include an examination of the major histocompatibility complex (MHC) and an outline of the laboratory practices involved in matching patients and potential donors.

Box 12.1 Haemopoiesis

Haemopoiesis takes place principally within the bone marrow where the pluripotent stem cells are continuously dividing. The pluripotent cells give rise to the myeloid and lymphoid stem cells. The progeny of the lymphoid stem cells develop, eventually, into the T and B lymphocytes and the natural killer cells, while the myeloid stem cells give rise to all the polymorphonuclear leucocytes, monocytes, red cells and platelets. The path in which the progeny develop is influenced by cytokines such as interleukin-3, granulocyte-macrophage colony stimulating factor (GM-CSF), granulocyte colony stimulating (G-CSF) and erythropoietin (EPO). These growth factors control the production of the individual groups of blood cell as they are required by the body. Cytokines which influence haemopoiesis are used in treating a number of transfusion-related syndromes. For example, the anaemia of patients in chronic renal failure may be treated with EPO, and patients with neutropenia following cancer chemotherapy may be given G-CSF.

12.2 SOME USEFUL DEFINITIONS

Haemopoietic stem cell transplants (HSCT) may be **autologous**, **allogeneic** or **syngeneic**, depending on the relationship between the donor and the recipient. When a patient is infused with his/her own stem cells, the transplant is autologous. An autologous transplant is given when the patient's HSC are harvested prior to treatments which would otherwise destroy their own, such as chemotherapy or radiotherapy. The HSC are stored during this process and infused back into the patient following treatment. Autologous transplants pose no risk of GVHD, because the transplant and the recipient are identical. If the transplant forms part of a treatment regime for cancer, care must be taken to ensure that no cancer cells are re-infused into the patient.

An allogeneic transplant is one obtained from another donor. The donor may be related, such as a sibling, or unrelated, provided a good 'match' is obtained. Allogeneic transplants pose a risk of GVHD. A syngeneic transplant is one obtained from an identical twin. Because identical twins have an identical genetic make-up, there is no risk of GVHD. However, such transplants are, obviously, quite rare.

Box 12.2 Terminology in organ and stem cell transplants

The terminology of transplants is somewhat different between HSCT and organ transplants. In the latter case, a transplant within one individual is termed an isograft or autograft, that between different individuals is termed an allograft (though it may also be called allogeneic), while the term syngeneic refers to transplants within a highly inbred strain of animal. Isografts or autografts are often used in plastic surgery as, for example, when healthy skin is used to treat a badly burned area. Syngeneic grafts are not relevant clinically while xenogeneic grafts (between different strains of animal) have been used as, for example, when a heart from a baboon has been implanted into a human. Transgenic grafts in humans are xenogeneic grafts from animals which have been genetically engineered to express human MHC antigens. Currently this work is experimental. Transgenic pigs have been developed to express human antigens but there is currently much debate about the ethics of transplanting organs from such animals into humans. Transgenic transplantation is most unlikely to be useful in haemopoietic cell transplantation where it is much more important to find histocompatible donors to prevent the development of GVHD.

12.3 CLINICAL SITUATIONS REQUIRING A HAEMOPOIETIC STEM CELL TRANSPLANT

Conditions for which HSCT is of value include immunodeficiency disorders, bone marrow failure, leukaemia and lymphoma, some solid tumours and some inherited disorders. These are discussed below.

Immunodeficiency. The first successful bone marrow transplant (BMT) took place in 1968 at the University of Minnesota. The treatment was given to a child with severe combined immunodeficiency disease (SCID), a primary immunodeficiency disorder resulting from defects in the lymphoid stem cells in the bone marrow. The child's sibling was the donor. Similarly, in 1973, the first successful BMT using an unrelated donor was also carried out on a child with SCID. Today, HSCT is used to treat a variety of primary immunodeficiencies as well as SCID and these include chronic granulomatous disease (CGD), Chédiak–Higashi syndrome, and Wiskott–Aldrich syndrome.

Bone marrow failure. A variety of conditions characterized by failure of the bone marrow may be treated with HSCT. These include aplastic anaemia, Fanconi's anaemia, paroxysmal nocturnal haemoglobinuria and congenital thrombocytopenia, myelodysplasia and pure red cell aplasia.

Leukaemias and lymphomas. The first use of BMT to treat leukaemia, using bone marrow from a histocompatible unrelated donor, was reported in 1979. Though the treatment itself was successful, the patient's leukaemia returned. Haemopoietic stem cell transplantation is, today, a commonplace procedure for the treatment of a variety of leukaemias and lymphomas, including acute myclogcnous and lymphoblastic leukaemias (AML and ALL), chronic myelogenous and lymphocytic leukaemia (CML and CLL), Hodgkin's and non-Hodgkin's lymphoma, multiple myeloma and juvenile myelomonocytic leukaemia. The rationale behind these treatments is to bring the patient into remission by high-dose chemotherapy or radiotherapy, which, while destroying cancer deposits in the bone marrow, also destroys the bone marrow itself. The patient is then 'rescued' with the HSCT. With an autologous transplant, the patient's own stem cells are obtained prior to transplant and stored until the conditioning regime is complete. Before transplantation, the sample may be 'purged' of cancer cells. This is possible if the cancer cells possess antigens not found on normal cells, in which case an antibody to the distinctive 'tumour-associated' antigen may be used to remove them. Further details of conditioning regimes are given below.

Solid tumours. HSCT is now commonly used in the treatment of a variety of solid cancers, especially those known to metastasize to bone. Total body irradiation of the patient after removal of the primary tumour and/or aggressive chemotherapy is used to destroy any cancer deposits in bone marrow. Patients are then given a HSCT to repopulate their bone marrow. This treatment has been used for patients with breast, renal, ovarian and testicular cancers, as well as small cell carcinomas of the lung and sarcoma.

Inherited metabolic disorders. A variety of inherited metabolic disorders are now treated with a HSCT. Examples include Hurler's syndrome, adreno-leucodystrophy, and haemoglobinopathies such as sickle-cell anaemia and β-thalassaemia major.

12.4 SOURCES OF HAEMOPOIETIC STEM CELLS FOR TRANSPLANT

Haemopoietic stem cells for transplant are derived from one of three sources, namely bone marrow, peripheral blood and umbilical cord blood. The most frequent source today is from peripheral blood. However, whatever the source, the stem cells are present in an abundance of other cells, including those which could bring about GVHD. Thus, it is necessary to identify the stem cells so that they can be purified and enriched prior to transplantation and, if necessary, to ensure the removal of T lymphocytes, the cells which bring about GVHD.

CD34 is a cell surface antigen which is expressed on human haemopoietic stem cells, both the pluripotent stem cells and the lineage-committed progenitor cells, such as the myeloid and lymphoid stem cells. The structure of CD34 consists of a core protein backbone which is highly glycosylated and includes sialic acid residues; the CD34 protein appears to promote adhesion to bone marrow stroma. CD34-positive cells account for approximately 1% of bone marrow cells and are rarely found in peripheral blood. Identification of the CD34 molecule on the haemopoietic stem cells has provided a means for their selection in order to enrich the transplant. This is usually achieved by a system which relies on the use of magnetic beads. The most common technique for isolating CD34+ cells is, first, to incubate the cells with a mouse monoclonal antibody to CD34. Following incubation, the cells are washed free of unbound antibody and mixed with polystyrene paramagnetic beads coated with an anti-mouse immunoglobulin antibody, to which they become bound. A magnetic field is used to remove the cells attached to the beads and the cells are released using a releasing reagent.

Enumeration of the CD34+ cells is achieved using a fluorescent antibody to CD34, followed by flow cytometry (see Chapter 13).

Bone marrow

As previously discussed, the history of HSCT began with the first successful BMT in 1968 and, until 1986, these were the most common type of HSCT in adults. Today, bone marrow accounts for less than 30% of HSCT in adults aged over 20 years, though it still accounts for around 60% of HSCT in those under 20 years of age. A BMT provides a source of stem cells, which migrate to the marrow of the patient and continue to produce immature blood cells, thus restoring normal haemopoiesis. Some clinicians may still choose bone marrow transplantation because the techniques have become well known and standardized over the last four decades. The marrow is harvested from various sites, particularly from both iliac crests of the hip bone whilst the donor is under general or local anaesthesia, the process taking about 1 hour. The aim is to collect sufficient cells to ensure speedy engraftment, usually a minimum of 3×10^8 nucleated bone marrow cells per kilogram of recipient body weight. This cell number contains approximately 2×10^6 CD34+ cells per kilogram of recipient body weight. The marrow is filtered to remove bone fragments. At this stage, the marrow may be infused into the recipient or it may require further processing. If there is a difference in ABO blood group between the donor and recipient, it is necessary to treat the marrow further to remove the red cells or contaminating plasma. Techniques are also available to remove T cells from the graft, which can reduce both the incidence and severity of GVHD. One method which may be used is to incubate the bone marrow cells with an antibody to CD3, a protein which is present in the membranes of all mature T lymphocytes. Addition of complement results in the lysis of these T cells.

Bone marrow stem cells are transfused into the patient intravenously, the progress is then monitored and transfusion support therapy given. The recipient may be given antibiotics because the patient is at risk of infection, at least until the marrow is engrafted and starts to produce blood cells. The recipient may also be given platelet and red cell transfusions to prevent bleeding and anaemia.

With an autologous transplant, marrow is harvested from the patient while in remission from the disease and this negates the need for a compatible donor. However, where the transplant is used to treat a malignancy such as leukaemia, it is necessary to 'purge' the marrow of any malignant cells, while preserving the viable haemopoietic stem cells. If the cancer cells carry a tumour-specific antigen, then they can be selectively killed using an antibody to the tumour-specific antigen in the presence of complement.

Peripheral blood stem cells (PBSC)

Until 1986, the major source of stem cells was bone marrow. Nowadays, peripheral blood stem cell transplantation (PBSCT) has largely replaced bone marrow as a source of autologous haemopoietic blood cells and outnumbers considerably the use bone marrow for allogeneic PBSCT in adults, but not in children. However, stem cells are rarely found in the circulation, and in order to increase the number of circulating stem cells for harvesting, the cells are 'mobilized' from the marrow into the peripheral blood by injection of G-CSF. This cytokine stimulates production of haemopoietic cells, in particular those cells which express the cell surface antigen CD34.

Reasons for the popularity of PBSCT include its ease of collection using the technique of **apheresis** and the reduced likelihood of the graft being affected by the presence of tumour cells from the existing disease. In addition, higher numbers of CD34+ cells can often be obtained and this is reflected in improved time to engraftment. It is now possible to isolate CD34+ cells to high levels of purity, thus significantly reducing the number of unwanted cells (see *Fig. 12.1*). The target dose is 5×10^6 cells per kg of body weight.

For transplants into children, PBSCT has produced poorer outcomes than with adults, and other sources, such as bone marrow or umbilical cord blood, are used in preference.

Box 12.3 Apheresis

Apheresis is a technique which is used for collection of specific blood components and has the advantage that blood is returned to the donor. This allows donations to be taken more frequently. In the collection of PBSC, a series of apheresis sessions take place over a few hours with minimum discomfort to the donor. Apheresis is also used for collection of blood components (see Chapter 9).

Human umbilical cord blood

A further rich source of haemopoietic stem cells is umbilical cord blood. The success of the umbilical cord blood transplantation in matched siblings, since its first use in 1988, has led to the establishment of cord blood banks in an attempt to increase further the unrelated donor pool. Umbilical cord

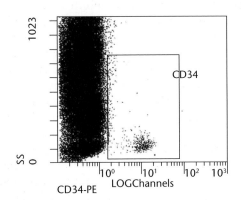

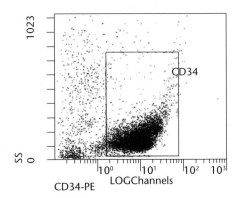

Figure 12.1

Scattergrams showing CD34 analysis of peripheral blood stem cells using flow cytometry. The vertical axis indicates side scatter and the horizontal axis indicates fluorescence intensity. Stem cells are characterized by low side scatter. Left: Pre-selection; CD34+ cells make up 0.7% of the cell population. Right: Post-selection; CD34+ cells make up 96% of the cell population. The CD34+ cells have been selected using magnetic activated cell sorting. Courtesy of T.F Carr, Royal Manchester Children's Hospital, Salford, UK.

blood is harvested with maternal consent, HLA typed (see later) and cryopreserved until required. Currently, around 30% of HSCT in children employ stem cells obtained in this way and results have shown a decreased incidence of GVHD. However, because only a small amount of blood is obtained from the umbilical cord and placenta, the technique is only suitable for children or small adults. The minimal dose of HSC obtained in this way is around 2.0×10^5 cells per kg of body weight.

Box 12.4 Cord blood banks

There is now an emerging industry involved in cord blood banking. These cord banks will, at a price, collect, test and preserve a baby's cord blood, for up to 20 years, for use in the future if the child falls ill. The most recent price quoted in the UK is around £1500 per donation.

  Private cord bank enterprises are controversial because, being stored for use by the individual, they may never be used, whereas a public cord bank, with donations voluntarily given, would ensure greater use of these cells. In addition, should the child have an inherited disorder, then he/she would need stem cells from a donor as their own would carry the defect.

12.5 PRE- AND POST-TRANSPLANT TREATMENTS

Processing and storage of haemopoietic stem cells

Depending on the source of the HSC, the volume of material may be reduced, for example by centrifugation in order to increase the cell concentration, either for transplant or for storage. Red cells are removed from ABO-incompatible bone marrow allografts by using sedimenting agents such as starch or dextran. CD34+ cells are enriched as described earlier. HSC may need to be stored for several days, especially if the patient is to be given conditioning treatment prior to transplantation or if more than one harvesting procedure is needed. This is achieved by a combination of irradiation and/or cytotoxic drugs and/or immunosuppression and may form part of the treatment for a malignant disease. It may therefore be necessary to store the harvested stem cells prior to infusion. Short-term (between 2 and 3 days) storage of bone marrow should be within a blood transfusion refrigerator at 4°C, whereas PBSC should be stored at 21–22°C with agitation to prevent platelet aggregation. Longer term storage requires cryopreservation in sealed containers with 10% dimethyl sulphoxide (DMSO) as a cryoprotective agent. Freezing is brought about in a programmed rate freezer which allows the cells to be cooled at the optimum rate for cell survival, normally approximately 1°C per minute. Storage is then in the gas or liquid phase of liquid nitrogen (approximately –176°C).

When cryopreserved HSC are required, the containers are removed from storage, placed in a sterile plastic bag and thawed rapidly at 37°C. A small sample is removed aseptically, for quality testing, and, if suitable, the cells are infused into the patient. The DMSO in the infusion is excreted, mainly via the lungs.

Conditioning treatment

All patients who are to receive a HSCT are given intensive therapy to kill their own bone marrow cells prior to transplant. This treatment includes toxic radiation therapy or chemotherapy and immunosuppression to prevent rejection of the graft and to prevent GVHD. Such high-intensity conditioning presents considerable toxicity to an already sick patient. More recently, reduced-intensity conditioning (RIC) prior to transplantation has been used, for example in patients who could not tolerate the high-intensity treatment.

Transfusion support post-transplant

Blood components such as red cells and platelets are needed for support therapy of a post-transplant patient (see *Box 12.5*). In some laboratories, these components may be irradiated with gamma rays as the process of irradiation prevents contaminating lymphocytes being activated. However, in the UK, irradiators are only found in large clinical centres and the National Blood Service laboratories. Another important consideration is the provision of blood components which are known to be negative for cytomegalovirus (CMV). This is because the patient is immunosuppressed and is highly prone to infection from sources which could include blood components. The transfusion of CMV-positive blood components may cause a recurrence of earlier CMV infection which has remained dormant in the patient.

Box 12.5 A patient with thalassaemia major

This case study concerns a young girl with thalassaemia major. Following conditioning, she was given a haemopoeitic stem cell transplant from a matched sibling on Day 0. The data table below shows her haemoglobin levels, leucocyte count and platelet count following the transplant:

Day	Hb (g dl⁻¹)	Leucocyte count (×10⁹ l⁻¹)	Platelets (×10⁹ l⁻¹)	Treatment
0	8.7	0.5	247	
1	9.8	0.11	110	
2	9.9	0.04	97	
3	9.6	0.03	91	
4	9.2	0.2	23	
5	8.9	0.03	70	
6	8.6	0.02	61	
7	8.4	0.04	50	
8	6.8	0.04	39	Red cells
9	7.1	0.05	45	Platelets
10	9.4	0.1	33	
11	8	0.15	32	Red cells and platelets
12	7.5	0.25	30	
13	9.6	0.25	6	Platelets
14	9.1	0.33	26	
15	10	0.73	25	Platelets
16	10.2	1.3	35	
17	9.9	1.88	29	
18	10.3	3.01	40	
19	10.6	2.1	36	
20	10.3	1.45	22	
21	9.5	2.83	23	
22	9.9	1.99	20	
23	9.4	1.24	26	
27	10.3	2.22	33	
34	10	1.65	87	
36	10.1	1.56	101	

Red cell transfusions were given on days 8 and 11. Hb levels approached normal (11 g dl⁻¹) following Day 16. Leucocyte counts, as expected, were initially very low (normal levels are 4–11 × 10⁹ l⁻¹) but began to pick up around Day 18. Platelets (normal levels 150–400 × 10⁹ l⁻¹) dropped dramatically and infusions were given where appropriate. By Day 36, these levels had begun to increase and approach the lower level of normal. The transplant was a success and the patient recovered without a major event.

12.6 PROBLEMS ASSOCIATED WITH HAEMOPOIETIC STEM CELL TRANSPLANTS

Problems which occur post-transplantation include infections, GVHD and possible rejection of the graft. In addition, patients may suffer a range of later complications related to the initial disease or to the use of steroids to suppress GVHD or rejection. Patients being given a transplant for the treatment of cancer may suffer a relapse. Other complications include iron overload due to multiple transfusions, endocrine problems, secondary malignancies and, rarely, viruses transmitted with transfusions.

Infections

The transplantation of HSC arises as a consequence both of the treatment itself and of the underlying disorder for which it provides a treatment. So, for example, patients requiring HSCT have an underlying immune deficiency either because they have a primary immunodeficiency, such as SCID, or because they have been treated with chemotherapy and/or radiation therapy which renders their bone marrow defective. Whatever the reason, the underlying immune deficit both pre and post transplant (until the transplant engrafts and the immune system is reconstituted), renders the patient highly prone to infections. During the immediate post transplant phase the patient must be kept in isolation in a room in which air is filtered to reduce fungal contamination. Antibiotics, antiviral and antifungal drugs may be given prophylactically and/or at the first sign of infection, such as fever. Intravenous immunoglobulin may also be given to protect against a broad spectrum of common bacteria. Following engraftment, patients may be prone to infection with cytomegalovirus (CMV), a particular risk with an allogeneic transplant. Emergence of CMV is monitored using PCR tests (Chapter 13) and antiviral drugs given if necessary.

Graft-versus-host disease

GVHD occurs under conditions in which a transplant recipient cannot reject the graft due to an underlying immune deficiency and the graft contains immunocompetent cells. T lymphocytes in the bone marrow respond to foreign MHC antigens on the recipient's cells and mount an immunological attack. This is therefore a problem when carrying out an allogeneic BMT and can be a serious limitation to stem cell transplantation. Around 50% of allogeneic transplants develop GVHD within the first 100 days post-transplant. In the acute form of GVHD, there is an extensive skin rash, which may progress to blistering and exfoliation, where the epithelial cells of the skin become necrotic and may be sloughed off. This may initially be confused with an allergic reaction, although transplant centres will be alert to such conditions. Similar occurrences in the intestine lead to diarrhoea, which may be profuse, watery and bloody. The liver and spleen may be affected, leading to enlargement of these organs and jaundice. Acute GVHD may result in the death of the patient. Chronic GVHD involves chronic desquamation of the skin and diarrhoea, spleen and liver enlargement and frequent secondary infections.

The incidence of GVHD may be reduced if T lymphocytes are removed from a graft prior to transplantation. However, such treatment of an allogeneic transplant being used to treat patients with leukaemia has been associated with a statistically significant increase in tumour relapse. The explanation appears to be that T cells in the graft may also be mounting an immune response against the tumour cells.

Patients who develop GVHD will need immunosuppressive therapy using drugs such as cyclosporin together with methotrexate or corticosteroids. Cyclosporin is a drug which targets the sensitized T cells attacking the host, while methotrexate inhibits cell division by inhibiting the enzyme dihydro-folate reductase, an enzyme required for the synthesis of purines and pyrim-idines, and therefore DNA. Corticosteroids are anti-inflammatory in action and are frequently used in combination with other immunosuppressive drugs.

Box 12.6 Transfusion-associated GVHD

GVHD may occur between 7 and 30 days following transfusion of whole blood containing small lymphocytes. It is now recognized that GVHD is a rare complication of transfusion of whole blood and blood products which contain residual leucocytes. It is particularly associated with transfusion of immunodeficient individuals (but not those with AIDS) and patients with aplastic anaemia, and may also occur following intrauterine transfusion of a foetus or transfusion of premature neonates whose immune systems are immature. GVHD has also been associated with transfusion of concen-trated red cells, platelets and fresh plasma, all of which may contain residual T lymphocytes. It is now recommended that such products be subjected to gamma irradiation (25–50 Gy) prior to trans-fusion to prevent any small lymphocytes from dividing (see Chapter 11). Plasma which has been frozen and thawed is safe to transfuse as any leucocytes which may have been present prior to freez-ing are destroyed by the freezing process. In addition, the process of leucodepletion renders blood products less likely to harbour residual leucocytes.

Rejection of the graft

Because a HSCT is usually given to patients who are immunodeficient, either through disease or through conditioning treatment, rejection is less of a problem than GVHD. However, patients receiving an allogeneic HSCT are treated with immunosuppressive drugs prior to transplant. Sometimes the pre-conditioning treatment is insufficient to prevent rejection of an allogeneic graft. This may occur where there are incompatibilities between the donor and the recipient or if the recipient is already sensitized to cells of the graft.

Graft rejection and GVHD are both caused by differences in major histo-compatibility antigens between the cells of the donor and the recipient.

12.7 THE MAJOR HISTOCOMPATIBILITY COMPLEX

Whether or not a graft is rejected (or whether GVHD occurs) depends on genetic differences between the donor and the recipient: the greater the genetic difference, the greater the chances of rejection. These genetic differ-ences relate to the expression of cell surface proteins encoded by a region of the genome called the **major histocompatibility complex** (MHC). The cell surface proteins encoded by the MHC are fundamentally important in the immune response because they 'present' foreign antigens to T lymphocytes (see Chapter 1). The role of these MHC molecules in all specific immune responses was demonstrated in 1973, some years after MHC molecules were shown to induce transplant rejection. Hence, their name reflects their involvement in transplant rejection, a somewhat artificial situation, rather than their role in the immune response generally.

The immune response is not directed against an entire MHC protein but merely against those regions which are different from the recipient's own MHC molecules. Transplantation scientists therefore tend to talk about MHC **antigens** rather than MHC proteins, because it is the antigens which are the main focus of interest. It is only necessary to remember that the antigens are regions of the MHC molecules to which antibodies bind.

Box 12.7 Rejection of solid transplants

The terms histocompatibility refers to whether a tissue will be accepted or rejected by an individual. MHC molecules were first discovered as a result of investigations by scientists such as Snell and Gorer into the genetics of the rejection of transplanted tumours in mice. They discovered a genetic region containing a complex set of genes coding for 'histocompatibility antigens'. This genetic region is known as the H2 region and is the murine MHC. The human MHC is known as the HLA system.

Rejection of organ transplants may take place within hours of the organ being attached to the blood supply of the recipient (hyperacute rejection) or, more usually, a few weeks after transplantation, which is known as acute rejection. Acute rejection is brought about primarily by T lymphocytes, and animals which have no T cells do not reject grafts. T lymphocytes (both CD4+ and CD8+) respond to the foreign histocompatibility antigens on the surface of the donated cells. The immune system produces cytotoxic T lymphocytes (CTL) directed against the foreign histocompatibility antigens on the grafted cells. CTL are capable of killing cells of the grafts directly or indirectly by releasing cytokines which attract and activate phagocytes, particularly monocytes and macrophages (see Chapter 1). In addition, sensitized CD4+ (helper) T lymphocytes respond by producing cytokines which activate a variety of non-specific cells to destroy the graft.

In a graft-versus-host response, the T lymphocytes in the graft respond to MHC molecules on the cells of the recipient. Thus, sensitized T lymphocytes, both CD4+ and CD8+, may attack any organ in the body, because MHC molecules are found on all the nucleated cells.

The MHC is a genetic region which codes for several different types of protein, classified as Class I, Class II and Class III. Class I MHC genes code for proteins found on the surface of all nucleated cells. They are integral membrane proteins which present antigens to CD8+ T lymphocytes (see Chapter 1). Class II MHC genes also code for integral membrane proteins but these are found on a restricted range of cells. Many of these cell types act as 'antigen-presenting cells' and present 'exogenous' antigen to CD4+ T lymphocytes.

Class III genes code for a variety of soluble proteins and are not relevant to this discussion. Examples of genes found within this region are those that code for the complement proteins C4 and C2 and the genes for different forms of tumour necrosis factor (TNF).

MHC Class I and II proteins

All Class I MHC proteins have a similar overall structure as shown in *Fig. 12.2*. This consists of a single polypeptide chain (RMM 45 000 Daltons) known as the alpha (α) chain. It is a transmembrane protein and has three distinct immunoglobulin-like domains, α_1, α_2 and α_3. This protein is always associated in the membrane with a smaller polypeptide known as β_2-microglobulin (β_2M; RMM 12 000 Da). This is not a transmembrane protein and is not encoded by the MHC but its expression seems to be necessary for the stability of the α chain in the membrane.

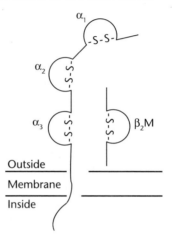

Figure 12.2
Diagram of an MHC Class I molecule. This consists of a single polypeptide chain (the α chain) and is found associated with the β_2-microglobulin chain, which is not encoded within the MHC.

Different Class I molecules are encoded at different genetic loci and these reflect fundamental differences between the overall amino acid sequences of the α chain. However, antigenic differences also occur between different forms of a Class I molecule encoded within a single genetic locus. These variations are due to allelic variations in genes at a particular locus. In this case, the differences in amino acid sequences which cause antigenic variations occur mostly in the α_1 and α_2 domains.

Class II proteins are made up of two polypeptide chains: an α chain (RMM 33 000 Da) and a β chain (RMM 28 000 Da). Both chains are encoded within the MHC. They are both transmembrane proteins with two immunoglobulin-like domains each (see *Fig 12.3*). There are several genetic loci encoding different Class II α and β chains within the Class II region of the MHC. In addition, there is considerable antigenic variation among Class II molecules specified at the same locus, which is accounted for by allelic variation. This will be discussed below in the context of the human MHC, which is otherwise known as **the HLA system** (see *Box 12.8*). The antigenic variation within Class II molecules specified at an individual locus is caused by amino acid sequence variations in the α_1 and β_1 domains.

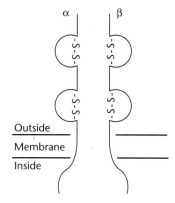

Figure 12.3
Diagram of an MHC Class II molecule. The MHC II molecule consists of two chains, the α and β chains, both encoded within the MHC.

Box 12.8 The HLA system

HLA stands for human leucocyte antigens. This is because they were first discovered from the observation, in 1958, that sera from patients who had received multiple blood transfusions would agglutinate leucocytes. Of course, it is now known that these antigens are not confined to leucocytes. Moreover, there are many leucocyte antigens which are not encoded by the HLA region. However, the human MHC is still known as the HLA system.

12.8 THE HLA SYSTEM

The HLA complex is found on the short arm of chromosome 6. A very simplified diagram of the HLA complex is shown in *Fig. 12.4*. The Class I region contains several genetic loci in each of which is a gene encoding a Class I α chain. The best-known loci are *HLA-A*, *HLA-B* and *HLA-C*, although there are others, such as *HLA-E*, *HLA-F* and *HLA-G*. The genes at each of these loci encode a different Class I protein. The protein products of these genes are isotypes, which means that the cells of the body express the products of each of these genes. In addition, because chromosomes

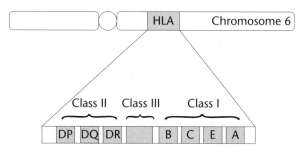

Figure 12.4
Schematic of the HLA system on chromosome 6.

come in pairs, the homologous chromosome 6 also contains the *HLA-A*, *-B* and *-C* loci. The genes within the loci on the two homologous chromosomes are alleles. This means that they are alternative forms of the genes, coding for proteins with slight variations in amino acid sequence (usually in the α_1 domain). These paired genes are co-dominant, which means that both alleles are expressed in cells. Therefore, nucleated cells in the body express two slightly different HLA-A proteins in their membranes as well as two different HLA-B proteins and two different HLA-C proteins.

Polymorphisms within the HLA system

In classical Mendelian genetics, a gene may exist in two allelic forms. These alleles have slightly different nucleotide sequences so that the proteins they encode will have similarly slight differences in amino acid composition. Depending on where these changes occur, the change of amino acid sequence may or may not affect the activity of the protein. However, even minor changes in amino acid composition can affect their immunogenicity.

As we have seen with blood groups described in earlier chapters, there are several genes which exist in many different allelic forms within a population, although an individual has only two of these alleles (one on each homologous chromosome). Such a system is said to be **polymorphic**. The MHC in higher vertebrates is one of the most highly polymorphic systems known and the HLA complex in man is no exception. So far, 506 alleles of the *A* gene, 851 alleles of the *B* gene and 276 alleles of the *C* gene have been discovered by sequencing the DNA encoding individual genes. Given that each individual has two of these alleles at each locus, it will be seen that the chances of individuals having the same 'set' of HLA genes is very small.

The Class II region

Within the Class II region are several genetic loci, the best known being *DP*, *DQ* and *DR* (see *Box 12.9*). Within each of these loci, there are genes encoding the α and the β chain of the Class II molecules. The situation is rather more complex than for Class I in that there may be more than one gene at each locus encoding the α and the β chains. For example, the *HLA-DR* region contains four genes for the HLA β chain. All of these β-chain products are expressed in a single cell, making the degree of variation much

---

Box 12.9 The Class II region of the HLA complex

Originally, the Class II region was known as the HLA-D region and was discovered, not serologically, but by genetic differences between small lymphocytes which would allow them to stimulate each other when cultured together in a technique known as the mixed lymphocyte reaction (MLR). Subsequently, anti-HLA sera were discovered which distinguished a number of proteins specified by genes at different loci within the HLA-D region. Thus, the loci within the Class II region were named HLA-DP, HLA-DQ and HLA-DR.

Table 12.3 Polymorphism of Class II genes

Gene	Codes for	Number of alleles*
HLA-DRA	α chain of HLA-DR	3
HLA-DRB	β chain of HLA-DR	559
HLA-DQA1	α chain of HLA-DQ	34
HLA-DQB1	β chain of HLA-DQ	81
HLA-DPA1	α chain of HLA-DP	23
HLA-DPB1	β chain of HLA-DP	126

*The alleles so named are based on sequence data obtained by sequencing the DNA; information has been obtained from www.anthonynolan.com/HIG/index.html.

higher. Like Class I, the Class II region also displays a high degree of polymorphism (see *Table 12.3* for details).

Discovery and naming of alleles

Alleles of HLA genes have been discovered in two different ways. Originally, new alleles were discovered when transplantation scientists discovered anti-sera with 'new' specificities against human leucocytes. However, the newer techniques of DNA sequencing, and the human genome project in particular, have allowed far more alleles to be discovered, even though antibodies against the products of these alleles have not necessarily been found. Thus, the number of alleles determined serologically is far less than those determined by DNA sequencing methods. New alleles are confirmed at major international workshops, which have met regularly since they were set up in the 1960s.

Historically, alleles at different loci were numbered as their existence was confirmed by scientists. Thus, for example, *HLA-B27* refers to an allele of the *HLA-B* gene. Complexities in this system have arisen, for example, when particular allelic variations occur together, due to nucleotide variations at different regions of the same gene. Each allele is now assigned a unique four, six or eight digit number in which the first two digits describe the type of antigen and subsequent numbers describe subtypes. Thus, for example, *HLA-DRβ1*0401* and *HLA-DRβ1*0404* are both subtypes of *DRβ1*04*.

HLA typing

Traditionally, tissue typing was carried out using serological methods. These use antibodies against individual HLA antigens to detect the corresponding antigens on the surface of peripheral blood lymphocytes (PBL). Today, serological methods are being used to complement DNA methods and the latter have been particularly useful in typing for genes within the Class II region.

Serological methods

The most common method is the lymphocytotoxicity assay. PBL are used when typing for Class I antigens and these are easily obtained from fresh whole blood. When typing for Class II antigens, B lymphocytes are used since T lymphocytes do not express Class II molecules. B lymphocytes can be obtained by enrichment from PBL by one of several methods.

For the lymphocytotoxicity assay, aliquots of freshly isolated, viable PBL or enriched B lymphocytes are pipetted into the wells of a 96-well micro-cytotoxicity plate (known as a Terasaki plate). Antibodies to HLA antigens are added, to individual wells. An antibody will bind to a small lymphocyte if the appropriate antigen is present on these cells. When complement is added, the cells are killed owing to activation of the classical pathway (see Chapter 3). Viability stains, which stain only dead cells, or which differentially stain dead and live cells, are added to each well and, thus, those wells in which an antibody has bound to an antigen will be seen to contain dead cells.

Traditionally, anti-HLA antibodies were obtained from the sera of multiparous women, i.e. women who have had several pregnancies, and from patients who had received multiple transfusions of whole blood. The specificity of these antibodies is first determined by screening them in a lymphocytotoxicity assay against a panel of cells of known HLA type. Monoclonal antibodies with known specificities are also used. For Class II typing, B lymphocytes are incubated with antisera to individual Class II antigens. Because most anti-HLA sera also contain antibodies to Class I antigens, these must be removed from the antiserum by incubating them with pooled platelets which also express Class I antigens. The platelets 'absorb' the anti-Class I antibodies and are removed by centrifugation.

Rabbit serum is used as a source of complement. Trypan blue and eosin Y are suitable viable stains. An alternative method is to stain the small lymphocytes with a fluorescent dye prior to testing. When the cells are killed, the dye leaks out and the cells are no longer visible with a fluorescence microscope. One popular method is to stain the cells with a mixture of acridine orange and ethidium bromide, both of which are fluorescent molecules. Acridine orange enters living cells and stains the nuclei green, while ethidium bromide enters dead cells and stains the nuclei red. A test is scored as strongly positive when more than 50% of the cells in a well are killed.

Crossmatching

A crossmatch is a test to detect pre-formed antibodies to graft antigens in the serum of a potential recipient. The test can be performed in a lymphocytotoxicity assay in which serum from the recipient is incubated with PBL from the donor. Complement is added and the viability of the cells tested as previously described. If donor cells are killed, it indicates that the recipient already has antibodies against graft antigens and is likely to be an unsuitable match.

DNA techniques

These techniques are based on the detection of DNA coding for an antigen rather than serological methods which detect the antigen itself. They have the advantage that smaller amounts of blood are required and the tests can be carried out on whole blood which has been stored frozen without cryoprotectant because, unlike serological assays, they do not require the presence of live cells.

DNA methods used for tissue typing include the detection of restriction fragment length polymorphisms (RFLPs) (see Chapter 13) and use of the polymerase chain reaction (PCR) to amplify an area of DNA which can then be probed with known sequences.

Variations of the PCR method include **sequence-specific oligonucleotide probing (SSOP)** and **sequence-specific priming (SSP)**. In SSOP, the gene of interest is amplified using primers which amplify all the common alleles of a particular locus. The PCR product is then probed with oligonucleotide sequences specific for particular alleles. In some laboratories, the individual oligonucleotides are attached to individual fluorescent microspheres. Incubation of the microspheres with the PCR product allows them to bind to any complementary HLA sequence. The microspheres, with bound PCR product, are then analysed by flow cytometry. SSOP is often used in initial typing of a donor or patient, whereas SSP is used for higher resolution typing, that is, typing to a four digit level. With SSP, the primers are specific for, and will only amplify, a particular allele. Hence, the product can be identified by the presence or absence of product.

HLA typing can only be undertaken in laboratories that have been accredited by the European Federation for Immunogenetics (EFI) or another organization using similar accreditation procedures. For an HSCT using an unrelated donor, both donor and recipient must be typed twice, using blood samples taken on two separate occasions. For an HSCT, the minimal requirements are for a complete match at the *HLA-A, -B, -C* and *-DRβ1* loci.

12.9 AVAILABILITY AND CHOICE OF DONOR

Donors of HSC for transplant are preferably related to the patient as this decreases the chance of GVHD. However, compatible related donors are available in only about 30% of cases and, increasingly, unrelated donors are used. The two main registries in the UK are the British Bone Marrow registry and the Anthony Nolan registry. The latter, for example, had 370 000 registered donors at the end of 2005. Both registries are linked to the International Bone Marrow Donors Worldwide (IBMDW), an internet organization with a potential 6 million donors throughout the world. However, new donors are always required locally to increase the number of HLA types available. The development of tissue typing using molecular techniques has reduced the risk of GVHD in HSCT recipients.

Factors affecting compatibility

The major difficulty in achieving a successful allogeneic HSCT comes from differences in the HLA system between donor and recipient. Differences in Class II HLA antigens are particularly relevant here. Problems of compatibility are increased when the HSC donor is unrelated to the patient requiring the transplant. The severity of GVHD is directly related to the degree of incompatibility, especially in the Class II region, and many patients do not have an HLA-identical sibling. In these circumstances, a combination of techniques is used at a serological, cellular and molecular level in an attempt to provide the most compatible transplant.

If an HSCT is the treatment strategy of choice, the initial approach is to HLA type the parents and siblings of the patient. Sometimes an identical HLA donor is found, in other cases a partial HLA mismatched relative may be an option. In mismatched donors, it is even more important to HLA type thoroughly, and again cellular and molecular techniques improve the likelihood of successful matching.

SUGGESTED FURTHER READING

Atkinson, K., Champlin, R., Ritz, J., Fibbe, W.E., Ljungman, P. and Brenner, M.K. (eds) (2004) *Clinical Bone Marrow and Blood Stem Cell Transplantation*, 3rd edn. Cambridge: Cambridge University Press.

Center for International Blood and Marrow Transplant Research (CIBMTR): http://www.ibmtr.org

European Group for Blood and Marrow Transplantation: http://www.ebmt.org

Grewal, S.S., Barker, J.N., Davies, S.M. and Wagner, J.E. (2003) Unrelated donor hematopoietic cell transplantation: marrow or umbilical cord blood? *Blood* **101**, 4233–4244.

Hoffbrand, A.V., Moss, P.A.H. and Pettit, J.E. (2006) *Essential Haematology*, 5th edn. Oxford: Blackwell Science.

Hughes-Jones, N.C., Wickramsinghe, S.N. and Hatton, C. (2004) *Lecture Notes on Haematology*. Oxford: Blackwell Publishing.

Loberiza, F.R. Jr, Serna, D.S., Horowitz, M.M. and Rizzo, J.D. (2003) Transplant center characteristics and clinical outcomes after hematopoietic stem cell transplantation: what do we know? *Bone Marrow Transplant* **31**, 417–421.

McKenna, D.H. and Clay, M.E. (2005) Haemopoietic stem cell processing and storage. In: *Practical Transfusion Medicine*, 2nd edn (eds M.F. Murphy and D.H. Pamphilon), Chapter 31. Oxford: Blackwell Publishing.

Pamphilon, D. (2004) Stem cell harvesting and manipulation. *Vox Sanguinis* **87**(S2), 20–25.

The Anthony Nolan Research Institute HLA Informatics Group: http://www.anthonynolan.org.uk/HIG/

The National Marrow Donor Program: at http://www.marrow.org/ABOUT/History/index.html

Williamson, L.M. and Navarrete, C.V. (2005) Immunomodulation and graft-versus-host disease. In: *Practical Transfusion Medicine*, 2nd edn (eds M.F. Murphy and D.H. Pamphilon), Chapter 18. Oxford: Blackwell Publishing.

SELF-ASSESSMENT QUESTIONS

1. Outline the difference between an **autologous** graft and an **allogeneic** graft.
2. What is meant by a 'histocompatibility antigen'?
3. State what feature of the immune system is responsible for (a) hyperacute rejection and (b) acute rejection of an organ transplant.
4. When may a blood transfusion cause graft-versus-host disease and how can this be avoided?
5. How do Class I and Class II MHC molecules differ in their tissue distribution?
6. How are tissues 'typed'?
7. List some disorders in which haemopoietic stem cell transplant has been of value.
8. Define the cells on which CD34 antigen is expressed.
9. List the benefits of umbilical cord blood stem cells compared with other options.
10. Give examples of problems concerning transfusion support in post-stem cell transplant patients.

CHAPTER 13

Applications of molecular and immunological techniques

Learning objectives
After studying this chapter you should be able to:

■ Describe the molecular techniques available for laboratory testing

■ Describe the application of DNA techniques to a variety of investigations in transfusion science

■ Describe the use of molecular techniques in HLA testing

■ Outline the principle of flow cytometry

■ Describe the applications of flow cytometry to the identification and quantification of membrane proteins

13.1   INTRODUCTION

The increased and now widely accepted use of molecular and immunological techniques has enhanced the body of knowledge in transfusion science. Serological methods which depend on the detection of haemagglutination, as described in Chapter 10, have their limitations in certain circumstances. For example, monitoring antibody levels in pregnant women gives only an indirect indication of the risk of haemolytic disease of the newborn (HDN) as antibody levels do not necessarily reflect the antigen status of the foetus. Another example is the problematic phenotyping of a recently multi-transfused patient due to the mixed population of red cells present. In addition, it can be difficult to phenotype red cells which are coated with IgG antibody. The highly specific blood group antigen typing performed on selected donors is only practical when a relatively small number of donors are tested for a relatively small number of antigens at any one time. Similarly, it may be difficult to provide the range of homozygous red cells required for investigating antibodies in patient's plasma in the laboratory screening tests. This is because some antigens are expressed so weakly on red cells that their detection by agglutination alone can be very variable. Another problem is that it is sometimes not possible to type cells for certain antigens because the availability of suitable antibodies is limited.

This chapter describes a selection of current applications of molecular and immunological techniques which have emerged to solve some of the problems described above.

13.2 MOLECULAR TECHNIQUES FOR THE IDENTIFICATION OF BLOOD GROUPS

The majority of genes encoding all of the blood group systems have now been sequenced and the molecular basis of most blood group antigens and many blood group phenotypes has been determined. This means that assays based on molecular techniques can be used in the clinical laboratory to overcome some of the limitations of serological methods.

Technology using the polymerase chain reaction

Molecular genotyping of individuals has become possible since knowledge of the sequence of a gene and the mutations responsible for the blood group antigen have become available. Allele-specific **probes**, or **primers**, may be specifically designed for use in the polymerase chain reaction (PCR) technique. PCR is a method of replicating a particular segment of DNA, which may then be analysed using gel electrophoresis. Probes (primers) are labelled nucleic acid fragments whose nucleotide sequences bind to known sequences within restriction fragments. They may be DNA or RNA in nature. PCR is based on the principle that DNA molecules have the ability to separate and be copied as strands of complementary DNA. The DNA segment is put through a series of cycles for its amplification (see *Box 13.1*).

Box 13.1 Amplification of DNA in the PCR

1. Denaturation of double-stranded DNA using heat.
2. Annealing: the hybridization of paired synthesized primers with a specific sequence of nucleotides to the complementary sequence of single-stranded DNA.
3. Using DNA polymerase, i.e. *Thermus aquaticus*, or *Taq*, to add free nucleotides in an order which is complementary to the template of single-stranded DNA. This extends the primers, and the new DNA, which is double-stranded, makes a new template for further amplification cycles. And so the process continues.

Laboratory application of PCR is usually coupled with two other techniques: allele-specific PCR (AS-PCR), which uses allele-specific primers for amplification as described, and restriction fragment length polymorphisms. Southern blotting is another technique used to visualize and identify the presence of particular genes in relation to known fragments of DNA (see *Box 13.2*).

Box 13.2 Southern blotting

The technique of Southern blotting was first described in 1975 by Dr Edmund Southern of Edinburgh. It uses DNA which is isolated and cut with restriction enzymes. The fragments are then sorted by size in a gel using electrophoresis, the smaller fragments migrating faster than the larger ones. The fragments are then transferred to a nylon or nitrocellulose membrane and the DNA is denatured into single strands. The sample of DNA is incubated with a probe which attaches to the complementary fragment being identified, i.e. a particular gene. The probe is labelled so it can be visualized, the method of visualization depending on the nature of the label used. Thus, the presence of a particular gene can be identified in relation to known fragments of DNA. Applications of molecular techniques are continually increasing and have significantly impacted on the quality of research and routine diagnostic testing in transfusion science in recent years.

Restriction fragment length polymorphisms

The basis of tests using restriction fragment length polymorphisms (RFLPs) is that DNA which varies in base sequence will produce different-sized fragments of DNA when 'cut' by restriction enzymes (bacterial endonucleases which cut DNA at specific base sequences). The fragments can be separated out by size using gel electrophoresis and transferred on to nylon membranes by blotting. The nylon membranes are then incubated with labelled DNA probes complementary to certain consensus sequences. This procedure will produce a banding pattern characteristic of certain alleles. This method requires a relatively large amount of DNA (5–10 µg).

Sequence-specific oligonucleotide probing

A number of techniques have been employed to amplify specific genes or regions. These include **sequence-specific oligonucleotide probing (SSOP)**, in which probes are made to anneal with sequences of DNA which are common to all the alleles being investigated, and **sequence-specific priming (SSP)** in which primers are designed to anneal with sequences of DNA which are specific to that allele/locus.

The source and quality of DNA

A common and easily available source of DNA is from leucocytes, but it is possible to obtain samples of DNA from any body cells (somatic cells). The lining of the mouth is an easily accessible source, for example. It is important to realise that the quality of DNA obtained from individuals is significant. Poor-quality DNA may decrease, or stop completely, the process of amplification. Other factors are necessary in controlling the process of amplification, for example the concentration of reagents used. Laboratory controls and experienced laboratory workers are essential components in establishing confidence that reactions are working properly.

13.3 APPLICATIONS OF MOLECULAR TECHNIQUES

The use of molecular techniques allows the possibility of matching blood donor antigen-negative status to that of chronically transfused patients. For instance, patients with sickle cell disease or other haemoglobinopathies will depend on regular, lifelong transfusions and are often stimulated to produce multiple blood group antibodies. This can make finding compatible donors increasingly difficult. Thus, the ability to match, as closely as possible, the donor antigen status to that of the patient is extremely important. Matching using conventional serology-based methods is difficult and time-consuming. There is now the possibility using molecular and microarray technology for the antigen-negative status of both donor and patient to be precisely matched. Such methods are both cost-effective and simple to perform. The genotyping of individuals for ABO blood group status by the detection of glycosyl transferases has provided a depth of knowledge about this blood group system, although it seems unlikely that molecular techniques will replace haemagglutination techniques in routine hospital laboratories.

Other applications for molecular techniques include the antigen typing of foetuses to identify those at risk of HDN when the mother has clinically significant antibodies. The foetal DNA can be detected in the maternal circulation, eliminating the need for potentially dangerous invasive procedures to obtain foetal blood. Quantitative DNA assays make it possible to accurately establish a patient's phenotype in the presence of transfused donor cells. This mixture of patient and donor red cells interferes with traditional serological typing methods. Phenotyping red cells which are coated in IgG antibody, using conventional serological methods, may cause false results (see Chapter 10). However, the bound IgG antibody does not interfere with the DNA assays. Molecular methods have proved valuable for establishing the zygosity of blood group genes, for instance when testing the husband of a pregnant woman who has blood group antibodies, and for establishing the zygosity of reagent red cells used for antibody identification by traditional serological methods. DNA assays enable the detection of weakly expressed antigens on red cells when serological methods give variable results and also the detection of certain antigens for which it is difficult to obtain the corresponding antibodies of sufficient potency, for example, antigens in the Dombrock system.

Microarray technology

The application of molecular biology to blood grouping has tremendous potential to change the way we perform tests in transfusion science and the use of microarray technology provides a mechanism to detect multiple parameters simultaneously. It can be used for rapid, accurate and complete genotyping of blood groups in both patients and donors. The principle of the technique involves the arrangement of synthetically prepared nucleotide sequences (probes), which determine blood group specificities, using a solid-phase microarray substrate. A microarray is an orderly arrangement of DNA probes, dispensed by accurate robotic techniques, on to glass slides which have been chemically treated with iminosilane. Thus, small amounts of single-stranded DNA fragments for each gene allele are fixed to the slide in a tightly spaced grid or 'array'. The addition of PCR-prepared material from the individual, and the resulting fluorescence shown when the complementary DNA (cDNA) corresponds to the DNA of the individual sample, can then be analysed electronically using computer software. A different gene allele is placed in each spot and the individual's single-stranded DNA is applied, having been made from mRNA by reverse transcriptase using fluorescently labelled nucleotides. This will hybridize with any complementary DNA on the microarray; excess DNA is rinsed away and the microarray is scanned for fluorescence. Each fluorescent spot represents a gene allele expressed on red cells. Whilst 'macroarrays' require 300 µl of blood sample and can be used to test hundreds of blood samples, microarrays require even less sample (200 µl) and can be used to test thousands of samples at a time. Thus, all regions of cDNA representing blood group polymorphisms can be detected. Sequencing of blood group genes has revealed that most alleles are due to single nucleotide polymorphisms (SNP), an example of which is shown in *Box 13.3* using blood group Kell as an example (see Chapter 7).

Box 13.3 Example of a SNP in the Kell blood group

The presence of methionine means that glycosylation does not take place in the KEL 1 blood group; however, substitution with the amino acid threonine does confer glycosylation.

Antigen	Point mutation	Exon	Amino acid substitution
KEL 1[K]	AAC CGA ATG CTG	6	Methionine
	Asn Arg Met Leu		
KEL 2[k]	AAC CGA ACG CTG	6	Threonine
	Asn Arg Thr Leu		

Limitations of DNA-based assays for blood groups

As can be seen from the examples above, the types of investigation for which DNA assays are most helpful are the highly complex situations which are less frequently encountered. Such cases would normally be sent to a specialized reference laboratory rather than be investigated in a routine hospital transfusion laboratory. Assays based on molecular techniques do not currently lend themselves to routine investigations such as ABO or Rh D typing of high numbers of patients or donors. In addition, such techniques can only be used to investigate antigen polymorphisms within blood groups, and are of no use in the characterization of blood group antibodies.

Molecular techniques detect grossly normal but unexpressed genes, which can lead to donors and patients being falsely blood group typed as antigen positive. It is not possible to analyse all polymorphisms, for example the high number of alleles encoding a single phenotype found in the ABO system, or a blood group in which the molecular basis has not yet been established (e.g. Vel and Lan). There is also a high probability that not all alleles (and therefore polymorphisms) in all ethnic populations have yet been identified and thus would continue to be undetected by current DNA assays.

13.4 FURTHER APPLICATIONS OF MOLECULAR TECHNIQUES

The use of RFLP and PCR has been applied to human leucocyte antigen (HLA) typing for transplant patients (see Chapter 12). Molecular biology techniques, which are based on the detection of DNA coding for an antigen, rather than serological methods, which detect the antigen itself, are currently being used to type for Class II HLA antigens.

PCR in HLA typing

PCR has been of value in the HLA typing of donors and recipients for organ transplantation. HLA typing is used to match stem cell and organ donors with recipients, and is particularly beneficial in HLA typing of patients with aplastic anaemia, who have very few leucocytes, or post-chemotherapy patients, whose low leucocyte count is the result of treatment. PCR is used to amplify an area of DNA by using primers specific for that particular region and the enzyme DNA polymerase. The method rapidly allows the production of multiple copies of a targeted area of DNA, as described earlier, and the amplified portions of HLA genes are analysed by electrophoresis, blotting and probing with short oligonucleotide probes which hybridize to sequences characteristic of particular HLA Class II alleles. PCR methods are useful because they require much less DNA initially. They can also be carried out on whole blood which has been stored frozen without cryoprotectant because, unlike serological assays, they do not require the presence of live cells.

PCR in the detection of viruses

PCR in transfusion laboratories is also known as nucleic acid testing, or NAT. The technique has been applied for the detection of small amounts of viral DNA in donor blood, samples of which are tested for viruses, such as hepatitis C virus, to prevent the transmission of disease to recipients of blood transfusions. It is particularly useful to confirm a negative result in the absence of antibody detection in the donor blood sample. Viral transmission of diseases by blood is rare, but it is important to detect and prevent their occurrence and molecular techniques have improved the rate of detection.

Pre-natal foetal genotyping

The application of molecular techniques to pre-natal Rh D genotyping of the foetus, in order to detect the possibility of HDN, has been highly successful. The basis of this uses the detection of the Rh D peptide chain by amplification of the exons involved in D antigen status (see Chapter 6). This is performed using a sample of the mother's blood, taken during the second trimester of pregnancy, from which cell-free foetal DNA can be identified and amplified using PCR. Early foetal Rh D genotyping using an Rh D PCR technique is highly sensitive and specific. This may have a future impact on the requirement of prophylactic anti-D for Rh D-negative mothers with an Rh D-negative foetus.

13.5 IMMUNOLOGICAL TECHNIQUES USING FLOW CYTOMETRY

The technique of flow cytometry has become increasingly popular as more laboratories have been able to access such equipment as flow cytometers and fluorescence-activated cell sorters. Flow cytometry can be defined as the measurement of physical or chemical characteristics of cells. In this process, cells are streamed in single file through a 'zone of analysis' which includes a laser light source and light detectors. As the cells move through the laser beam, light is scattered in different directions. Light collected at 90° to the original axis measures side scatter. Simultaneously, a second detector measures forward scatter, i.e. light scattered in a forward direction up to 10° from the incident beam. The forward scatter is sensitive to the surface characteristics of the cell, whereas side scatter is more sensitive to the granularity of a cell (see *Fig. 13.1*). In addition to forward and side scatter, cells can be stained with fluorescent antibodies to antigens which are characteristic of a cell population. As the cells are illuminated in the laser beam, they fluoresce, and this fluorescence is picked up by further detectors, using appropriate filters. Thus, cell populations can be identified by fluorescence intensity following staining with appropriately labelled monoclonal antibodies (see *Fig. 13.2*).

The monoclonal antibodies, pre-labelled with fluorochromes, are, nowadays, easily obtained from commercial sources, although the process of attachment of fluorochromes to antibodies is not difficult. Examples of commonly used fluorochromes are fluoroscein isothiocyanate (FITC), which produces an apple-green fluorescence, phycoerythrin (PE), which produces red fluorescence, and thiazole orange.

Results obtained when fluorescing cells are analysed in the flow cytometer are displayed on an oscilloscope and computer software is used to transmit results for further translation. The operator may choose to select a cell population by the electronic process of 'gating'. Only the data for the selected cell type are then considered in the results.

The technique can also be adapted to look for particular cellular characteristics such as antibodies or membrane proteins, examples of which are described further below.

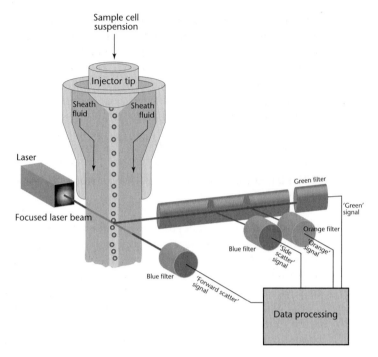

Figure 13.1
Principle components of a flow cytometer. The sheath fluid is hydrodynamically focused by adjusting the flow rate so that a single file of cells passes the light source. Approximately 1000 'events' per minute can be counted.

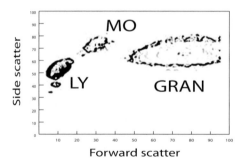

Figure 13.2
Oscilloscope bitmap showing the separation of three types of leucocytes in lysed blood. This example shows the separation of monocytes (MO), lymphocytes (LY) and granulocytes (GRAN).

Platelet antibodies

Platelet-associated antibodies may be detected in patients with immune thrombocytopenic purpura, platelet allo-antibodies may be formed in response to a transfusion of platelet concentrate, and platelet-bound immunoglobulin may be detected in neonatal allo-immune thrombocytopenia (described in Chapter 8). Some knowledge of platelet antigens is required in order to understand the application of flow cytometry for their detection. A brief explanation of human platelet antigens is shown in *Box 13.4*. Platelet antibodies may be induced in patients who lack a specific antigen on their own platelets. Platelet membrane proteins present surface **CD markers** (see *Boxes 13.4* and *13.5*). Commercially available monoclonal antibodies, to which fluorochromes are attached, are added to the patient or donor platelet sample. The selected CD marker for the platelet membrane protein, if present, will bind to the corresponding monoclonal antibody. The platelet sample is injected into the flow cytometer, which is gated specifically for platelets, and the resulting intensity of fluorescence is analysed. In order to demonstrate the presence of platelet antibodies, an indirect technique is used based on the same principle as the indirect antiglobulin test for red cell antibodies. Platelets are harvested from donors and incubated with the patient's serum. After a washing phase, the sample is incubated with FITC-conjugated anti-IgG. The resulting immunofluorescence indicates the presence of platelet allo-antibodies. Platelets are also analysed by size and granularity using the facility of forward scatter (FSC) and side scatter (SSC) of the light source, respectively. The technique of flow cytometry by platelet indirect immunofluorescence test is known as FC-PIFT.

Box 13.4 Common human platelet antigen types (HPA) and relevant CD markers

System	Antigen	Glycoprotein	CD
HPA-1	HPA-1a	GPIIIa	CD61
	HPA-1b		
HPA-2	HPA-2a	GPIbα	CD42b
	HPA-2b		
HPA-3	HPA-3a	GPIIb	CD41
	HPA-3b		
HPA-4	HPA-4a	GPIIIa	CD61
	HPA-4b		
HPA-5	HPA-5a	GPIa	CD49b
	HPA-5b		
HPA-15	HPA-15a	–	CD109
	HPA-15b		

Flow cytometry can also be used to detect HLA-specific antibodies, which may significantly affect the success of an organ transplant and bring about hyperacute rejection (see Chapter 12).

Detection of Rh D-positive foetal cells

Some examples of the use of flow cytometry include the detection and quantification of specific cellular membrane proteins which are specific for

---

Box 13.5 CD markers on human leucocytes

The term 'CD' stands for 'cluster of differentiation'. The term originated when, shortly after the first development of monoclonal antibodies by Kohler and Milstein in 1975, scientists began to develop monoclonal antibodies to human leucocytes. One reason for doing this was to identify different populations of cells by the identification and detection of characteristic cell surface markers. Thus, the monoclonal antibody OKT3 was found to identify human T lymphocytes. As more and more monoclonals were developed, it became clear that several monoclonals produced by different laboratories were, in fact, detecting the same antigen, even though they were not necessarily binding to the same epitope (see Chapter 1) on that protein. In 1982, the first Human Leucocyte Differentiation Antigens (HLDA) workshop was held to try to bring order to this situation. They introduced the CD classification, which identified clusters of antibodies with similar patterns of binding to leucocytes at different stages of differentiation. Thus, CD4+ cells are all stained by a CD4 cluster of antibodies which identify this marker on helper T lymphocytes. The last HLDA workshop was held in 2004; the number of CD markers now stands at 350 (see http://www.hlda8.org/). The workshops now refer to human cell differentiation molecules (HCDM) rather than HLDA, as it is recognized that these molecules are not necessarily found exclusively on leukocytes.

---

minor cell populations. The detection and quantification of Rh D-positive foetal cells in a blood sample from a mother who is Rh D negative, in order to assess the extent of foeto-maternal haemorrhage, is more accurately performed by flow cytometry than by the frequently used Kleihauer–Betke stain. In this situation, foetal red cells differ from maternal red cells as they contain foetal haemoglobin (HbF) and are Rh D-antigen positive. The maternal blood sample is first stained to identify the foetal red cells. The sample is incubated with monoclonal antibodies to either Rh D antigen or intracellular HbF, combined with fluorescent markers such as FITC and PE. The detection of Rh D-positive foetal cells may be achieved by direct or indirect methods. The indirect method involves two incubations: the first incubates the maternal blood with either anti-D or anti-HbF. In this phase, anti-D or anti-HbF will bind to the foetal cells. The second incubation uses a secondary antibody such as anti-human globulin immunoglobulin directed at the anti-D or anti-Hb, conjugated with a fluorochrome. Flow cytometry detects very low numbers of foetal cells in maternal blood, thus the extent of foeto-maternal haemorrhage can be accurately quantified.

Identification of transfused donor red cells

In the process of blood transfusion, it is sometimes necessary to distinguish transfused red cells from the patient's own, autologous, red cells. For this, the presence of an antigen on the transfused red cells which is absent from the recipient's own red cells is required. The corresponding monoclonal antibody to the selected antigen, and fluorescent marker, are incubated with the patient's red cells. Thus, the transfused red cells can be identified and quantified by the fluorescence intensity produced by the detection of the antigen (see *Box 13.6*).

Box 13.6   The use of flow cytometry to detect two cell populations in a blood sample

The following case describes a child suffering from a rare congenital disease known as Blackfan–Diamond anaemia. The clinical consequences are a lack of red cell development in the bone marrow (hypoplasia) resulting in a gradual, persistent anaemia. The child, who was diagnosed aged 7 years, was transfused regularly with red cell concentrates to prevent the symptoms of severe anaemia due to a very low haemoglobin and red cell count. His blood group was typed for ABO, Rh and Kell status using serological (agglutination) tests. He appeared to be either group O, Rh DCee, kk or group O Rh Dccee, kk, The serology results showing a 'mixed field' of agglutination, i.e. some agglutinated red cells and some free red cells. Initially he was transfused with O Rh-negative (dce) blood. As he required regular transfusions, it was necessary to establish his exact blood type with regard to Rh D, C, c, E and e, and Kell antigens to prevent antibodies being induced in response to donor blood. Unfortunately, the child had already been transfused with donor blood prior to establishing his correct blood type. This meant that his blood was a mixture of donor red cells and his own red cells, and therefore it was impossible to find out his own blood type, particularly whether he possessed the c or C antigen. Using flow cytometry, it was possible to distinguish transfused red cells from the child's own red cells. In order to do this, at least one antigen must be present on the child's red cells that is different from the donor cells. In this case it was the D antigen, as he was Rh D positive but had been transfused with Rh D-negative blood. Two-colour immunofluorescence was used: an IgG anti-D for green fluorescence, conjugated to FITC, and a biotin-conjugated IgM anti-C for red fluorescence. A sample of the child's blood was washed and incubated with these antibodies and fluorescence intensity was measured by flow cytometry. Thus, anti-D demonstrated green fluorescence, whilst anti-C showed red fluorescence. The results showed that the D antigen-positive cells, which were the child's, were also positive for the C antigen. This clearly differentiated the child's cells from the dce (rr) donor red cells. The case demonstrates the use of flow cytometry to distinguish two antigens simultaneously, using two different colours. The child could then be transfused with the correct blood type.

Umbilical cord or peripheral blood haemopoietic stem cells (HSC) may need to be identified in order to assess the quality of a donation for engraftment. The number of haemopoietic stem cells in a stem cell harvest can be quantified using a monoclonal antibody corresponding with the CD34 antigen, as HSC are known to be CD34 positive (see Chapter 12). A further use, post-stem cell transplant, is in monitoring the appearance of a new red cell population in the patient's peripheral blood, and disappearance of the patient's (autologous) red cells. The 'purging' of donated HSC to remove unwanted leucocytes or malignant cells is described in Chapter 12.

Assessing the quality of leucodepletion

The detection of residual leucocytes in donor blood is performed using flow cytometry. This is undertaken in order to assess the effectiveness of the filtration process for leucodepletion, an essential step in reducing the risk of prion transmission, e.g. variant Creutzfeldt–Jakob disease, and other leucocyte-related infections. Leucodepletion is also useful in reducing a number of leucocyte-related complications. For more details, see Chapter 11.

Bacterial contamination of platelet concentrate

The requirement for storage at room temperature raises the problem of sterility for platelet concentrates. A number of techniques are under development to address this issue and one assay has been developed by the German Red Cross in collaboration with a commercial company. The assay utilizes thiazole orange to stain bacterial nucleic acid. The stained bacteria then can be detected by their fluorescence using flow cytometry.

13.6 CONCLUSION

This brief review of techniques and their applications is by no means exhaustive and new applications of existing techniques are continually being developed. Furthermore, emerging technologies are increasing in many areas of transfusion science with the result that knowledge for the transfusion scientist is ever expanding.

SUGGESTED FURTHER READING

Daniels, G., Finning, K., Martin, P. and Soothill, P. (2004) Fetal blood group genotyping from DNA from maternal plasma: an important advance in the management and prevention of haemolytic disease of the fetus and newborn. *Vox Sanguinis* **87**, 225–232.

Daniels, G. (2004) Molecular blood grouping. *Vox Sanguinis* **87**(S1), S63–S66.

HLDA Workshop: http://www.hlda8.org

Kennedy, G.A., Shaw, R., Just, S., *et al.* (2003) Quantification of feto-maternal haemorrhage (FMH) by flow cytometry: anti-fetal haemoglobin labelling potentially underestimates massive FMH in comparison to labelling with anti-D. *Transfusion Medicine* **13**, 25–33.

Lee, A.H. and Reid, M.M. (2000) ABO blood group system: a review of molecular aspects. *Immunohematology* **16**(Special Millennium Issue), 1–6.

Reid, M.E. (2003) Applications of DNA-based assays in blood group antigen and antibody identification. *Transfusion* **43**, 1748.

Ridgwell, K. (2004) Genetic tools PCR and sequencing. *Vox Sanguinis* **87**(S1), S6–S12.

Robb, J.S., Roy, D.J., Ghazal, P., Allan, J. and Petrik, J. (2006) Development of non-agglutination microarray blood grouping. *Transfusion Medicine* **16**, 119–129.

Westhoff, C.M. (2006). Molecular testing for transfusion medicine. *Current Opinions in Hematology* **13**, 471–475.

SELF-ASSESSMENT QUESTIONS

1. List the molecular techniques which have been used in transfusion research.

2. Give two examples comparing DNA-based assays with alternative techniques.
3. Describe the use of PCR to determine the genotype of a foetus.
4. Describe the benefit of molecular techniques in HLA testing.
5. Describe the principles of flow cytometry.
6. List three fluorochromes which may be used in flow cytometry.
7. Define the term 'cluster of differentiation'.
8. Describe three applications of flow cytometry in identifying or quantifying membrane proteins.

Answers to self-assessment questions

Chapter 1

1. The two work very closely together: products of specific immunity affect the non-specific responses and *vice versa*.
2. Specificity and immunological memory.
3. They are secreted by cells and they affect other cells by binding to cell surface receptors and stimulating transmembrane events.
4. Neutrophils – blood; monocytes – blood; macrophages – found throughout the body; collectively phagocytes are found everywhere and this is important because foreign material can enter at any site in the body.
5. The process brings plasma and neutrophils into an area of tissue damage in which infection might occur.
6. When it is prolonged, for example, by a chronic infection.
7. On the whole, humoral immunity deals with extracellular pathogens while cell-mediated immunity deals with intracellular pathogens.
8. A bacterium is made up of many different proteins, glycoproteins, lipoproteins, etc., each of which is immunogenic.
9. From the Bursa of Fabricius where they develop in birds.
10. They all have different cell surface receptors for an epitope.
11. In specific immunity, small lymphocytes exposed to an immunogen first proliferate before they differentiate. Specific immunity depends on cell division.

Chapter 2

1. (a) IgG; (b) IgM; (c) IgE; (d) IgA.
2. Immunoglobulins are classified according to the type of heavy chain they possess.
3. IgG is used for passive immunization because it has a relatively long half-life.
4. IgM has μ heavy chains whereas IgG has γ heavy chains. IgM is a pentameric structure whereas IgG is monomeric.
5. The variable regions of heavy chains of immunoglobulins from different plasma cells always have a different amino acid sequence. The sequence of amino acids in all antibodies of the same class remains the same in the constant region.
6. To activate complement; to control transfer across the placenta; to activate phagocytes; to bind to large granular lymphocytes.
7. Steric, hydrophobic, hydrogen bonds, ionic interaction, Van Der Waal's forces.
8. Affinity describes the strength of binding of a single binding site for an epitope. Avidity describes the strength of binding of antibodies to an immunogen.
9. By binding to receptors for IgG on phagocytes and stimulating phagocytosis; by activating complement – some complement proteins opsonize immunogens, others attract neutrophils and some stimulate inflammation.

Chapter 3

1. IgM is the most efficient antibody at activating complement.
2. The activation of complement involves a number of enzymic stages which cause amplification in the system.
3. Newly activated complement proteins often have a transient hydrophobic binding site which allows them to bind to the cell membrane of the antibody-coated cell.
4. An anaphylatoxin stimulates degranulation of mast cells and basophils. The histamine released

causes vasodilation and inflammation. Chemotactic factors for neutrophils and eosinophils attract these cells into the site of complement activation.

5. Complement levels may be assessed by looking at the ability of the serum to lyse sheep red cells coated with sub-agglutinating levels of antibody.

6. Complement may be inactivated by heating to 56°C for 30 minutes.

7. Calcium and magnesium ions are needed for complement activation. EDTA is a chelating agent and effectively removes these ions from a solution to which it is added.

Chapter 4

1. A codon is a triplet of bases, for example, adenine, guanine and cytosine, which code for a specific amino acid or act as a stop/start signal.

2. An allele refers to a gene which exists in alternate forms at the same locus of homologous chromosomes.

3. The DNA organic bases are adenine, guanine, cytosine and thymine.

4. Inheritance via autosomal chromosomes.

5. Independent assortment takes place during the separation of chromatids in meiosis. It occurs when genes of homologous chromosomes are situated too far apart to be inherited together, or in genes of non-homologous chromosomes. Dependent assortment occurs in genes on the same chromosome where the loci, i.e. position on the chromosome, are close. Thus, the genes move together to the newly formed sex cells during the procedure of 'crossing over' of chromatids in meiosis.

6. The role of tRNA is to transfer amino acids from the cell pool to the ribosomes where they attach to the opposite base pairs of the codon in mRNA, thus forming a polypeptide chain.

7. Three types of mutation are:
   (1) silent mutation: this is when an amino acid is substituted for another but it has no evident effect on the phenotype;
   (2) missense mutation: this is when substitutions of bases result in a change in the amino acid sequence, which may result in the formation of an abnormal protein;
   (3) frameshift mutation: these occur due to insertion or deletion of bases which cause changes in the codon, resulting in a change to the reading frame.

8. There are many examples of nucleotide substitution to choose from; see *Table 4.1* for a list. One specific example is seen in the Duffy blood groups Fy^a and Fy^b where the amino acid glycine is substituted by asparagine.

9. The products of genes are proteins. Blood group antigens are either defined by proteins, such as the membrane proteins of the Rh blood groups, or they are defined by enzymes (also proteins) which attach substances to the red cell membrane.

Chapter 5

1. The *ABO* gene consists of seven exons, found on chromosome 9. The alleles for *A* and *B* differ by seven nucleotides and encode four different amino acid substitutions, at positions 176, 235, 226 and 268 of the enzyme transferases.

2. The enzymes are: α1,2-fucosyl transferase for blood group O, *N*-acetylgalactosaminyl tranferase for blood group A and D-galactosyl transferase for blood group B.

3. L-fucose.

4. The *FUT1* gene encodes α1,2-fucosyl transferase in tissues derived from the embryonic mesoderm and is responsible for the presence of H antigen on red cells, denoted by L-fucose. Absence of this gene leads to 'Bombay'-type blood groups; despite the *ABO* genotype no A- or B-determining sugars are found on the red cells. An absence of the *FUT2* gene results in a lack of secretion of A, B or H sugars in body fluids.

5. Group A = *N*-acetyl-galactosamine; group B = D-galactose; group O = L-fucose.

6. See *Table 5.5*.

7. See *Table 5.1*.

8. Subgroups A_1, A_2 and A_x are produced as a result of a defective *N*-acetyl-glycosyl tranferase which is less effective both in the quantity and quality of A sugars being attached to the red cell precursor chain.

9. They are 'cold' antibodies, reacting best at room temperature, usually 16–22°C.

Chapter 6

1. *Cis* effect – when the gene for the D antigen is on the same chromosome as a gene for the C or E antigens, the expression of C and E antigens may be depressed. *Trans* effect – the depressed expression of the D antigen which is due to the

presence of the gene for the C antigen on the opposite chromosome.

2. Two loci exist: the *RHD* gene, which forms the RHD polypeptide expressing the D antigen, and the *RHCE* gene, which forms the RHCE polypeptide expressing the C/c and E/e antigens.

3. The five major antigens of the Rh system are: D, C, c, E and e.

4. Rh immune antibodies attach to red cells at 37°C. The antiglobulin test or enzyme-treated red cells are used for their detection.

5. Patients who are partial D types (e.g. category D^{VI}) may produce antibodies against the missing D epitopes if transfused with normal Rh D-positive blood. It is therefore safer to type them as Rh D-negative and transfuse them with Rh D-negative donor blood. Babies who are partial D types do not normally immunize their Rh D-negative mothers due to the low immunogenicity of the partial D. It is therefore not considered important to detect these partial D types.

6. The gene arrangements are D and C and e on one chromosome (R$_1$) and D and c and E on the other (R$_2$). The genotype using Fisher notation is thus R$_1$R$_2$.

Chapter 7

1. Le^a, Le^b, P$_1$, P^k, I and i. Also, A, B and H antigens are carbohydrate structures.

2. Antigens which are protein structures are MNSs, Lutheran, Kell, Duffy, Kidd and Rh antigens.

3. I and i antigens differ in that I is a branched carbohydrate series and i is a linear carbohydrate structure. Furthermore, I is expressed on the red cells of adults, whilst i is expressed on the red cells of infants. The i antigen is converted to the branched form by an enzyme as the individual matures.

4. Complement-binding antibodies include: P system antibodies, anti-I, antibodies of the Duffy and Kidd system, and some antibodies of Le^a and Le^b blood groups.

5. Glycophorin A of the MN system acts as a receptor for *P. falciparum*; also Duffy antigens form the site of attachment for *P. vivax*.

Chapter 8

1. Warm haemolytic anaemia is caused by antibodies which cause haemolysis of red cells at 37°C,

i.e. body temperature. These antibodies may be connected with viral infections, tumours or immune diseases such as SLE.

2. Cold haemolytic anaemia occurs when antibodies are produced which attach to red cells at lower temperatures, from approximately 4°C to 28°C. They may arise in response to infection (e.g. *M. pneumoniae* or Epstein–Barr virus).

3. Haemolysis occurs due to damage to the red cell membrane. This causes leakage of haemoglobin, which is then further degraded. Haemolysis may be intravascular, taking place in the blood vessels, or extravascular, occurring in the reticulo-endothelial system. Free haemoglobin may be detected in the plasma or in the urine. The breakdown of haemoglobin results in raised levels of bilirubin in the circulation. Extravascular mechanisms also exist.

4. There are three types of drug-induced haemolytic anaemia:
   (a) antibodies induced due to the presence of the drug, which form a complex with the drug and attach to the red cells;
   (b) membrane modification: antibodies formed due to proteins on the red cell surface, which are induced by the presence of the drug;
   (c) antibodies formed in response to the attachment of the drug onto the surface of the red cells.

5. Kernicterus refers to the yellow pigmentation of bilirubin in the brain. Bilirubin is a breakdown product of haem, which is produced in blood vessels when there is haemolysis. Very high levels result in damaged brain tissue. The levels of bilirubin may be reduced either by phototherapy with ultraviolet light, or by exchange transfusion of blood.

6. Anti-D immunoglobulin should be given to all Rh-negative pregnant women, either during the pregnancy, within 82 hours of childbirth, in any adverse event resulting in loss of the foetus, or post-amniocentesis or other trauma which may have caused leakage of foetal cells into the mother.

7. The Kleihauer–Betke stain is based on the principle that foetal haemoglobin is resistant to elution from the red cells in an acid environment whereas adult (maternal) haemoglobin is not. This results in pink foetal cells which may be counted to estimate the number present in the mother's circulation.

8. Acute autoimmune thrombocytopenic purpura, chronic thrombocytopenic purpura and allo-immune thrombocytopenic purpura.
9. The term 'purpura' refers to a skin rash seen in patients with a reduced number of circulating platelets. It occurs due to tiny haemorrhages into the skin from the underlying capillaries.

Chapter 9

1. Red cell concentrate, platelets, fresh frozen plasma and cryoprecipitate.
2. Massive blood loss (together with a volume expander), anaemia, pre- and post-surgery, during surgery.
3. Platelets should be stored at room temperature and constantly agitated.
4. 2,3-DPG lowers the affinity of haemoglobin for oxygen so that the oxygen is released to the tissues.
5. Leucocytes are viral transmitters, especially cytomegalovirus; they present the antigens of the HLA system; they produce cytokines; and they may carry prions.
6. Filtering, which removes viruses by the process of leucodepletion; heat treatment to 80°C for 72 hours; and use of chemicals such as methylene blue, or solvent/detergent treatment to inactivate viral replication.
7. Haemorrhage due to low levels of coagulation factors, for example, consumption of factors due to disseminated intravascular coagulation, or impaired synthesis due to liver disease.
8. Recombinant factor VIII is selected as it is free from human, viral or vCJD contamination.

Chapter 10

1. Temperature, pH, ionic strength, antigen and antibody concentration.
2. Inadequate washing of the red cells prior to the addition of AHG regent. Faulty reading technique leading to disruption of agglutinates.
3. The enzymes remove negative surface charge from the red cell by removing glycophorins.
    a. This reduction in charge allows the red cells to approach one another more closely, so that the small IgG antibodies can span the gap between adjacent red cells.
    b. By removing proteins from the red cell surface, enzymes may make hidden antigen sites more accessible to antibody.

c. Similarly they may increase the mobility of proteins within the membrane, allowing for antigen clustering and the formation of multiple intercellular bridges.
d. Enzymes reduce hydration at the red cell surface, which favours antigen/antibody binding.
e. They promote the formation of irregular protrusions from the red cells. These protrusions exhibit less repulsive force due to their highly curved surfaces.

4. Ionic bonds, hydrogen bonds, hydrophobic bonds, van der Waal's forces, randomization of water.
5. Due to the electrical charges involved, on the red cells and in the saline, the zeta potential keeps the red cells apart by a minimum distance of approximately 20 nm. IgM antibodies have a distance between binding sites of approximately 30 nm and so can bridge the gap between adjacent red cells. The binding sites of IgG antibodies are only approximately 12 nm apart and so cannot bridge the gap between red cells suspended in saline.

Chapter 11

1. HBV by testing for HBsAg (surface antigen); HCV by testing for anti-HCV antibodies and HCV nucleic acid testing; HIV 1 and 2 by testing for antibodies; HTLV 1 and 2 by testing for antibodies; syphilis by *Treponema pallidum* haemagglutination assay testing for antibodies.
2. Clerical error at the time of sample collection from the patient, collection of donor blood from the laboratory or at the time of transfusion, leading to transfusion of the blood to the wrong patient.
3. All reactions should be reported to the hospital transfusion laboratory in the first instance. Then, bacterial or viral infections should be reported to the local transfusion centre as soon as possible. All adverse reactions resulting from the transfusion of blood components are reported to the Medicines and Healthcare products Regulatory Agency and the Serious Hazards of Transfusion group.
4. By gamma irradiation of the red cell or platelet component to inactivate the donors leucocytes.
5. Iron overload.
6. Post-transfusion purpura may occur as a result of anti-platelet antibodies in the patient which

destroy the transfused donor platelets, or due to sequestration of the patient's platelets in the spleen in association with transfused microaggregates.

7. The risks of viral transmission may be minimized by careful selection of donors, testing of donors and inactivation of viruses in plasma fractions by heat and/or chemical treatment of the product.

8. The patient's post-transfusion sample should be tested for ABO and Rh D type. It should be screened for clinically significant red cell antibodies. A direct antiglobulin test should be performed and the sample re-crossmatched against all available donor units (used and unused).

9. Leucodepletion prior to storage removes the risk of reactions due to the cytokines and histamine released from leucocytes during storage.

Chapter 12

1. An autologous graft is transferred within an individual. An allogeneic graft is transferred between two individuals.

2. A histocompatibility antigen is a cell surface protein which stimulates rejection of a graft.

3. (a) Antibodies; (b) T lymphocytes.

4. When it contains viable lymphocytes and is given to an immunodeficient individual or a premature neonate. Leucodepletion prevents transfusion-associated GVHD.

5. Class I molecules are found on all nucleated cells. Class II molecules are restricted to antigen-presenting cells.

6. (a) Serologically, using anti-HLA antibodies.
   (b) By RFLP or PCR, using oligonucleotide probes.

7. Leukaemia and some other malignancies, aplastic anaemia, congenital immunodeficiency, some inherited enzyme deficiency disorders.

8. Pluripotent and lineage-committed stem cells.

9. Freely available (subject to maternal permission); do not require cytokine treatment (as for PBSCT) or operation (bone marrow).

10. Blood and blood product transfusions must be irradiated to prevent transfusion of viable lymphocytes and the development of GVHD. Blood and products should be negative for CMV, even if the patient is already CMV-positive.

Chapter 13

1. Polymerase chain reaction; allele-specific PCR, restriction fragment length polymorphisms; sequence-specific oligonucleotide probing.

2. (a) In pre-natal assessment of the risk of haemolytic disease of the newborn. This is because the antibody levels (or titre) do not necessarily reflect the antigen status of the foetus.
   (b) The detection of small amounts of viral nucleic acid in donor blood which is screened for viruses, such as hepatitis C virus, to prevent the transmission of disease to recipients of blood transfusions. It is particularly useful to confirm a negative result in the absence of antibody detection, and most donors test as negative. Thus, we are attempting to detect a very occasional positive result in donor blood, which may only possess a tiny amount of nucleic acid if the infection is latent.

3. This is performed using a sample of the mother's blood, from which the foetal DNA can be identified and amplified using PCR. The RhD peptide chain, the presence of which indicates that the foetus is Rh D positive, can be detected by amplification of the exons involved in encoding the D antigen.

4. DNA-based tests are useful for the HLA typing of patients with few leucocytes such as aplastic anaemia or post-chemotherapy patients. These tests require much less DNA initially and tests can also be carried out on whole blood which has been stored frozen without cryoprotectant because they do not require the presence of live cells, unlike serological assays.

5. See *Figure 13.1*. The sheath fluid is hydrodynamically focused by adjusting the flow rate so that a single file of cells passes the light source. Approximately 1000 'events' per minute can be counted as cells pass the light source. Fluorescence can be incorporated to further identify and quantify cells using specific flurochomes. Fluorochromes are bound to monoclonal antibodies which have been raised against numerous antigens.

6. Fluoroscein isothiocyanate (FITC), phycoerythrin (PE), thiazole orange.

7. A set of characteristic cell surface markers which can be identified using monoclonal antibodies bound with fluorochromes and detecting fluorescence.

8. (a) Differentiation of foetal cells from maternal cells in assessing the extent of foetal-maternal haemorrhage. This may be using anti-D to detect Rh D-positive foetal cells and Rh D-negative maternal cells, or it may be by determining the presence of foetal haemoglobin using anti-HbF.

    (b) To assess the quality of the filtration process for leucodepletion of donor blood. A monoclonal antibody against a CD antigen for leucocytes is used; thus, any leucocytes present would be detected by fluorescence.

    (c) The identification of platelet antigens in order to type a patient or donor so that the inducement of platelet antibodies by platelet tranfusion is avoided.

Index

Page numbers in roman numerals refer to the colour plates